Advances In Organ-Specific PET Instrumentation and Their Clinical and Research Applications

Editors

HABIB ZAIDI
SULEMAN SURTI
ABASS ALAVI

PET CLINICS

www.pet.theclinics.com

Consulting Editor
ABASS ALAVI

January 2024 • Volume 19 • Number 1

ELSEVIER

1600 John F. Kennedy Boulevard ● Suite 1800 ● Philadelphia, Pennsylvania, 19103-2899

http://www.pet.theclinics.com

PET CLINICS Volume 19, Number 1
January 2024 ISSN 1556-8598, ISBN-13: 978-0-443-18402-4

Editor: John Vassallo (j.vassallo@elsevier.com)
Developmental Editor: Varun Gopal

PET Clinics (ISSN 1556-8598) is published quarterly by Elsevier Inc., 360 Park Avenue South, New York, NY 10010-1710. Months of issue are January, April, July, and October. Periodicals postage paid at New York, NY, and additional mailing offices. Subscription prices per year are $288.00 (US individuals), $100.00 (US students), $304.00 (Canadian individuals), $100.00 (Canadian students), $306.00 (foreign individuals), and $140.00 (foreign students). For institutional access pricing please contact Customer Service via the contact information below. To receive student and resident rate, orders must be accompanied by name of affiliated institution, date of term, and the signature of program/residency coordinator on institution letterhead. Orders will be billed at individual rate until proof of status is received. Foreign air speed delivery is included in all Clinics subscription prices. All prices are subject to change without notice. POSTMASTER: Send address changes to PET Clinics, Elsevier Health Sciences Division, Subscription Customer Service, 3251 Riverport Lane, Maryland Heights, MO 63043. **Customer Service: 1-800-654-2452 (U.S. and Canada); 314-447-8871 (outside U.S. and Canada). Fax: 314-447-8029. E-mail: journalscustomerservice-usa@elsevier.com (for print support); journalsonlinesupport-usa@elsevier.com (for online support).**

Reprints. For copies of 100 or more of articles in this publication, please contact the Commercial Reprints Department, Elsevier Inc., 360 Park Avenue South, New York, NY 10010-1710. Tel.: 212-633-3874; Fax: 212-633-3820; E-mail: reprints@elsevier.com.

PET Clinics is covered in MEDLINE/PubMed (Index Medicus).

Contributors

CONSULTING EDITOR

ABASS ALAVI, MD, MD (Hon), PhD (Hon), DSc (Hon)
Professor of Radiology and Neurology, Director of Research Education, Division of Nuclear Medicine, Department of Radiology, Hospital of the University of Pennsylvania, Perelman School of Medicine, University of Pennsylvania, Philadelphia, Pennsylvania, USA

EDITORS

HABIB ZAIDI, PhD
Professor, Geneva University Hospital, Division of Nuclear Medicine and Molecular Imaging, Geneva, Switzerland

SULEMAN SURTI, PhD
Research Professor, Department of Radiology, Perelman School of Medicine, University of Pennsylvania, Philadelphia, Pennsylvania, USA

ABASS ALAVI, MD, MD (Hon), PhD (Hon), DSc (Hon)
Professor of Radiology and Neurology, Director of Research Education, Division of Nuclear Medicine, Department of Radiology, Hospital of the University of Pennsylvania, Perelman School of Medicine, University of Pennsylvania, Philadelphia, Pennsylvania, USA

AUTHORS

AMER ALASSI, MD
Mallinckrodt Institute of Radiology, Washington University, St Louis, Missouri, USA

MAGDELENA S. ALLEN, BA
Department of Radiology, A. A. Martinos Center for Biomedical Imaging, Massachusetts General Hospital, Department of Physics, Massachusetts Institute of Technology

PAOLO CASTELLUCCI, MD
Nuclear Medicine, IRCCS Azienda Ospedaliero-Universitaria di Bologna, Bologna, Italy

CIPRIAN CATANA, MD, PhD
Associate Professor, Department of Radiology, Harvard Medical School, A. A. Martinos Center for Biomedical Imaging, Charlestown, Massachusetts, USA

STEFANO FANTI, MD
Nuclear Medicine, IRCCS Azienda Ospedaliero-Universitaria di Bologna, Bologna, Italy

ANDREA FAROLFI, MD
Nuclear Medicine, IRCCS Azienda Ospedaliero-Universitaria di Bologna, Bologna, Italy

AMY M. FOWLER, MD, PhD
Associate Professor, Department of Radiology, University of Wisconsin-Madison School of Medicine and Public Health, Department of Medical Physics, University of Wisconsin Carbone Cancer Center, University of Wisconsin-Madison, Madison, Wisconsin, USA

ALBERT GJEDDE, MD, DSc
Department of Clinical Medicine, Translational Neuropsychiatry Unit, Aarhus University, Denmark; Department of Neuroscience, University of Copenhagen, Denmark

ANTONIO J. GONZALEZ, PhD
Instituto de Instrumentación para Imagen Molecular (I3M), Centro Mixto CSIC, Universitat Politècnica de València, Valencia, Spain

ANDREA GONZALEZ-MONTORO, PhD
Instituto de Instrumentación para Imagen
Molecular (I3M), Centro Mixto CSIC,
Universitat Politècnica de València, Valencia,
Spain

SRILALAN KRISHNAMOORTHY, PhD
Department of Radiology, Perelman School of
Medicine, University of Pennsylvania,
Philadelphia, Pennsylvania, USA

JAE SUNG LEE, PhD
Department of Nuclear Medicine, Seoul
National University College of Medicine,
Brightonix Imaging Inc, Seoul, South Korea

MIN SUN LEE, PhD
Environmental Radioactivity Assessment
Team, Nuclear Emergency and Environmental
Protection Division, Korea Atomic Energy
Research Institute, Daejeon, South Korea

ADRIENNE L. LEHNERT, PhD
Research Scientist, Department of Radiology,
University of Washington, Seattle, Washington,
USA

RICCARDO MEI, MD
Nuclear Medicine, IRCCS Azienda
Ospedaliero-Universitaria di Bologna,
Bologna, Italy

KANAE K. MIYAKE, MD, PhD
Department of Advanced Medical Imaging
Research, Graduate School of Medicine, Kyoto
University, Kyoto, Japan

ROBERT S. MIYAOKA, PhD
Research Professor, Department of Radiology,
University of Washington, Seattle, Washington,
USA

YUJI NAKAMOTO, MD, PhD
Department of Diagnostic Imaging and Nuclear
Medicine, Graduate School of Medicine, Kyoto
University, Kyoto, Japan

CRISTINA NANNI, MD
Nuclear Medicine, IRCCS Azienda
Ospedaliero-Universitaria di Bologna,
Bologna, Italy

MICHELE SCIPIONI, PhD
Department of Radiology, Harvard Medical
School, A. A. Martinos Center for Biomedical
Imaging, Charlestown, Massachusetts,
USA

SULEMAN SURTI, PhD
Research Professor, Department of Radiology,
Perelman School of Medicine, University of
Pennsylvania, Philadelphia, Pennsylvania,
USA

AHMED TAHA, MD
Mallinckrodt Institute of Radiology,
Washington University, St Louis, Missouri,
USA

YUAN-CHUAN TAI, PhD
Associate Professor, Departments of
Radiology, and Biomedical Engineering, and
Electrical and System Engineering,
Washington University, St Louis, Missouri,
USA

MIWAKO TAKAHASHI, MD, PhD
Institute for Quantum Medical Science,
National Institutes for Quantum Science and
Technology, Inage-ku, Chiba, Japan

SODAI TAKYU, PhD
Institute for Quantum Medical Science,
National Institutes for Quantum Science and
Technology, Inage-ku, Chiba, Japan

HIDEAKI TASHIMA, PhD
Institute for Quantum Medical Science,
National Institutes for Quantum Science and
Technology, Inage-ku, Chiba, Japan

DEAN F. WONG, MD, PhD
Mallinckrodt Institute of Radiology,
Departments of Radiology, Psychiatry,
Neurology, and Neuroscience, Washington
University, St Louis, Missouri,
USA

TAIGA YAMAYA, PhD
Institute for Quantum Medical Science,
National Institutes for Quantum Science and
Technology, Inage-ku, Chiba, Japan

Contents

This review article focuses on PET detector technology, which is the most crucial factor in determining PET image quality. The article highlights the desired properties of PET detectors, including high detection efficiency, spatial resolution, energy resolution, and timing resolution. Recent advancements in PET detectors to improve these properties are also discussed, including the use of silicon photomultiplier technology, advancements in depth-of-interaction and time-of-flight PET detectors, and the use of artificial intelligence for detector development. The article provides an overview of PET detector technology and its recent advancements, which can significantly enhance PET image quality.

Dedicated brain PET scanners are optimized to provide high sensitivity and high spatial resolution compared with existing whole-body PET systems, and they can be much cheaper to produce and install in various clinical and research settings. Advancements in detector technology over the past few years have placed several standalone PET, PET/computed tomography, and PET/MR systems on or near the commercial market; the features and capabilities of these systems will be reviewed here.

Dedicated breast PET scanners currently have a spatial resolution in the 1.5 to 2 mm range, and the ability to provide tomographic images and quantitative data. They are also commercially available from a few vendors. A review of past and recent advances in the development and performance of dedicated breast PET scanners is summarized.

This article summarizes the evolution of dedicated prostate PET instrumentation. It starts by introducing prostate cancer, as well as the most common diagnostic and staging methods that are used in the clinics. Then, it describes the key aspects of PET detectors and their assembly in full PET scanners highlighting the most suitable geometries for prostate examination, and a review on the existing prostate dedicated PET. Finally, the next steps for extending the use of PET in the daily diagnose, staging, and image-guided biopsy of patients with prostate cancer are discussed.

Biomedical research has long relied on small-animal studies to elucidate disease process and develop new medical treatments. The introduction of in vivo functional imaging technology, such as PET, has allowed investigators to peer inside their subjects and follow disease progression longitudinally as well as improve understanding of normal biological processes. Recent developments in CRISPR, immuno-PET, and high-resolution in vivo imaging have only increased the importance of small-animal, or preclinical, PET imaging. Other drivers of preclinical PET innovation include new combinations of imaging technologies, such as PET/MR imaging, which require changes to PET hardware.

Organ-specific PET scanners continues to draw interest for their high-resolution imaging capability that is unmatched by whole-body PET/computed tomography (CT) scanners. The virtual-pinhole PET concept offers new opportunities in PET system design, allowing one to mix and match detectors of different characteristics to achieve the highest performance such as high image resolution, high system sensitivity, and large imaging field-of-view. This novel approach delivers high-resolution PET images previously available only through organ-specific PET scanner while maintaining the imaging field-of-view of a clinical PET/CT scanner to see the entire body.

Compton imaging has been recognized as a possible nuclear medicine imaging method following the establishment of SPECT and PET. Whole gamma imaging (WGI), a combination of PET and Compton imaging, could be the first practical method to bring out the potential of Compton imaging in nuclear medicine. With the use of such positron emitters as ^{89}Zr and ^{44}Sc, WGI may enable highly sensitive imaging of antibody drugs for early tumor detection and quantitative hypoxia imaging for effective tumor treatment. Some of these concepts have been demonstrated preliminarily in physics experiments and small animal imaging tests with a developed WGI prototype.

PET technology has immense potential for furthering understanding of the brain and associated disorders, including advancements in high-resolution tomographs and hybrid imaging modalities. Novel radiotracers targeting specific neurotransmitter systems and molecular markers provide opportunities to unveil intricate mechanisms underlying neurologic and psychiatric conditions. As PET imaging techniques and analysis methods continue to be refined, the field is poised to make significant contributions to personalized medicine for more targeted and effective interventions. PET instrumentation has advanced the fields of neurology and psychiatry, providing insights into pathophysiology and development of effective treatments.

Breast-specific positron imaging systems provide higher sensitivity than whole-body PET for breast cancer detection. The clinical applications for breast-specific positron imaging are similar to breast MRI including preoperative local staging and neoadjuvant therapy response assessment. Breast-specific positron imaging may be an alternative for patients who cannot undergo breast MRI. Further research is needed in expanding the field-of-view for posterior breast lesions, increasing biopsy capability, and reducing radiation dose. Efforts are also necessary for developing appropriate use criteria, increasing availability, and advancing insurance coverage.

The diagnosis of prostate cancer (PCa) is usually based on transrectal or transperineal biopsies (from 12 to 24 samples) in most cases after the performance of a dedicated MRI and/or transrectal ultrasound. A small-dedicated PET scanner could improve spatial resolution and increase sensitivity, allowing a precise detection and location of the PCa foci, thus allowing an image-guided biopsy. In this short review, we will focus our attention on the potential application of a dedicated prostate PET scanner and on the prototype that has been already assembled for this purpose.

PET CLINICS

SERIES OF RELATED INTEREST

Advances in Clinical Radiology
Available at: Advancesinclinicalradiology.com
MRI Clinics of North America
Available at: MRI.theclinics.com
Neuroimaging Clinics of North America
Available at: Neuroimaging.theclinics.com
Radiologic Clinics of North America
Available at: Radiologic.theclinics.com

THE CLINICS ARE AVAILABLE ONLINE!
Access your subscription at:
www.theclinics.com

PROGRAM OBJECTIVE
The goal of the *PET Clinics* is to keep practicing radiologists and radiology residents up to date with current clinical practice in positron emission tomography by providing timely articles reviewing the state of the art in patient care.

TARGET AUDIENCE:
Practicing radiologists, radiology residents, and other health care professionals who provide patient care utilizing radiologic findings.

LEARNING OBJECTIVES
Upon completion of this activity, participants will be able to:
1. Review advances and significant progress in understanding how breast cancer behaves.
2. Discuss PET instrumentation and its clinical applications.
3. Recognize PET detector technology's desired properties and its crucial role in determining PET image quality.

ACCREDITATION
The Elsevier Office of Continuing Medical Education (EOCME) is accredited by the Accreditation Council for Continuing Medical Education (ACCME) to provide continuing medical education for physicians.

The EOCME designates this journal-based CME activity for a maximum of 10 *AMA PRA Category 1 Credit*(s)™. Physicians should claim only the credit commensurate with the extent of their participation in the activity.

All other health care professionals requesting continuing education credit for this enduring material will be issued a certificate of participation.

DISCLOSURE OF CONFLICTS OF INTEREST
The EOCME assesses conflict of interest with its instructors, faculty, planners, and other individuals who are in a position to control the content of CME activities. All relevant conflicts of interest that are identified are thoroughly vetted by EOCME for fair balance, scientific objectivity, and patient care recommendations. EOCME is committed to providing its learners with CME activities that promote improvements or quality in healthcare and not a specific proprietary business or a commercial interest.

The planning committee, staff, authors, and editors listed below have identified no financial relationships or relationships to products or devices they or their spouse/life partner have with commercial interest related to the content of this CME activity:
Jae Sung Lee, PhD; Min Sun Lee, PhD; Ciprian Catana, MD, PhD; Michele Scipioni, PhD; Srilalan Krishnamoorthy, PhD; Suleman Surti, PhD; Antonio J. Gonzalez, PhD; Andrea Gonzalez-Montoro, PhD; Kothainayaki Kulanthaivelu, BCA, MBA; Adrienne L. Lehnert, PhD; Michelle Littlejohn; Robert S. Miyaoka, PhD; Yuan-Chuan Tai, PhD; Taiga Yamaya, PhD; Hideaki Tashima, PhD; Sodai Takyu, PhD; Miwako Takahashi, MD, PhD; Ahmed Taha, MD; Amer Alassi; Albert Gjedde, MD; Paolo Castellucci, MD; Riccardo Mei, MD; Andrea Farolfi, MD; Cristina Nanni, MD; Habib Zaidi, PhD; Abass Alavi, MD, PhD (HON); Magdelena Suriano Allen

The planning committee, staff, authors, and editors listed below have identified financial relationships or relationships to products or devices they or their spouse/life partner have with commercial interest related to the content of this CME activity:
Stefano Fanti, MD: Speaker/Consultant: Advanced Accelerator Applications, A Novartis Company, Astellas, Amgen, Bayer, Debiopharm, GE Healthcare, Janssen, Novartis, Telix

Amy M. Fowler, MD, PhD: Advisor/Researcher: GE Healthcare

Kanae K. Miyake, MD, PhD: Researcher: Shimadzu Corporation

Yuji Nakamoto, MD, PhD: Researcher: Shimadzu Corporation

Dean F. Wong, MD, PhD: Researcher: Eisai, Anavex, Roche; Consultant: Engrail Therapeutics

UNAPPROVED/OFF-LABEL USE DISCLOSURE
The EOCME requires CME faculty to disclose to the participants:
1. When products or procedures being discussed are off-label, unlabelled, experimental, and/or investigational (not US Food and Drug Administration [FDA] approved); and
2. Any limitations on the information presented, such as data that are preliminary or that represent ongoing research, interim analyses, and/or unsupported opinions. Faculty may discuss information about pharmaceutical agents that is outside of FDA-approved labelling. This information is intended solely for CME and is not intended to promote off-label use of these medications. If you have any questions, contact the medical affairs department of the manufacturer for the most recent prescribing information.

TO ENROLL

To enroll in the *PET Clinics* Continuing Medical Education program, call customer service at 1-800-654-2452 or sign up online at http://www.theclinics.com/home/cme. The CME program is available to subscribers for an additional annual fee of USD 254.00

METHOD OF PARTICIPATION

In order to claim credit, participants must complete the following:
1. Complete enrolment as indicated above.
2. Read the activity.
3. Complete the CME Test and Evaluation. Participants must achieve a score of 70% on the test. All CME Tests and Evaluations must be completed online.

CME INQUIRIES/SPECIAL NEEDS

For all CME inquiries or special needs, please contact elsevierCME@elsevier.com

Preface

Innovations in Organ-Specific PET Instrumentation: Quo Vadis

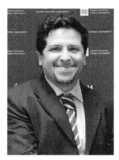 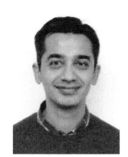 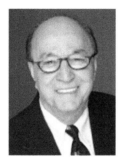

| Habib Zaidi, PhD | Suleman Surti, PhD | Abass Alavi, MD |

Editors

This is a thrilling time for innovative molecular imaging instrumentation in the era of precision medicine. The bulk of research to date in PET instrumentation focused on development of high-temporal-resolution detector modules to achieve the best performance from time-of-flight technology, improving the sensitivity through increasing the axial coverage, and integration of solid-state photodetectors (eg, Silicon photomultipliers) on (digital) clinical PET scanners. Significant research and development efforts were spent on improving the performance of dedicated systems during the last decade in both academic and corporate settings, resulting in the design of a number of systems suitable for clinical and research applications. Key examples include PET scanners dedicated to high-resolution imaging of the brain, breast, and prostate, in addition to preclinical systems intended for biomedical research.

In the current issue, we asked experts in the field to share their views, opinions, and experience with organ-specific PET scanners and their clinical applications. Prospects and suggestions for further research are also discussed. The contribution, by Lee and Lee, "Advancements in PET Detectors: From Silicon Photomultipliers Technology to Artificial Intelligence Applications," focuses on reviewing recent advances in PET detector modules and solid-state photodetectors, including the potential of artificial intelligence–powered algorithms in improving performance. The article by Allen

and colleagues, "New Horizons in Brain PET Instrumentation," provides a comprehensive review of dedicated brain PET scanners developed in academic and corporate settings with particular emphasis on innovations in instrumentation and conceptual designs carried out during the last decade. The conceptual design of PET scanners constructed for imaging other organs, such as the breast and prostate, is comprehensively reviewed in the two articles, "Advances in Breast-PET Instrumentation," by Krishnamoorthy and Surti, and "Developments in Dedicated Prostate PET Instrumentation," by Gonzalez and Gonzalez-Montoro. The contribution by Lehnert and Miyaoka, "Innovations in Small-Animal PET Instrumentation," summarizes advances in high-resolution small-bore PET systems intended for small-animal imaging. A thorough appraisal of the potential of a virtual-pinhole PET insert in enhancing spatial resolution through zoom-in imaging capability implemented on existing commercial clinical whole-body PET scanners is provided in the article by Tai, "High-Resolution Imaging Using Virtual-Pinhole PET Concept." The basic concept of whole-gamma imaging that combines PET and Compton imaging and is expected to potentially provide a practical approach for clinical implementation of Compton imaging in nuclear medicine is reviewed in the article by Yamaya and colleagues, "Whole-Gamma Imaging: Challenges and Opportunities." Potential clinical applications of the above

PET Clin 19 (2024) xi–xii
https://doi.org/10.1016/j.cpet.2023.09.004
1556-8598/24/© 2023 Published by Elsevier Inc.

reviewed dedicated systems (brain, breast, and prostate) are reviewed in the articles, "Transforming Neurology and Psychiatry: Organ-Specific PET Instrumentation and Clinical Applications," by by Taha and colleagues, "Clinical Applications of Dedicated Breast PET," by Fowler and colleagues, and "Potential Clinical Applications of Dedicated Prostate PET," by Castellucci and colleagues.

The development of advanced organ-specific PET instrumentation and related image reconstruction algorithms, as well as associated clinical applications, has been very fast and thrilling, and there is every reason to trust the field will move forward even more rapidly in the future. There is no scarcity of challenges and opportunities for advanced PET instrumentation and innovative clinical applications nowadays. We hope that, in this limited space, we were able to provide a flavor of recent advances in dedicated PET instrumentation and potential applications in clinical and research settings. We would like to thank the authors who contributed these articles and hope that the whole issue will be a valuable resource to readers.

CONFLICT OF INTEREST/DISCLOSURES

The editors have no conflicts of interest to disclose.

Habib Zaidi, PhD
Geneva University Hospital
Division of Nuclear Medicine and
Molecular Imaging
CH-1211 Geneva, Switzerland

Suleman Surti, PhD
University of Pennsylvania
Department of Radiology
Philadelphia, PA, USA

Abass Alavi, MD
University of Pennsylvania
Department of Radiology
Philadelphia, PA, USA

E-mail addresses:
habib.zaidi@hcuge.ch (H. Zaidi)
surti@pennmedicine.upenn.edu (S. Surti)
abass.alavi@pennmedicine.upenn.edu (A. Alavi)

Advancements in Positron Emission Tomography Detectors
From Silicon Photomultiplier Technology to Artificial Intelligence Applications

Jae Sung Lee, PhD[a,b], Min Sun Lee, PhD[c],*

KEYWORDS

- Positron emission tomography • Scintillation detector • Depth-of-interaction • Time-of-flight
- Silicon photomultiplier • Cherenkov light • Artificial intelligence

KEY POINTS

- PET image quality is determined by various physical and technical factors but the most critical one is PET detector technology. This is because PET detectors provide the essential information necessary for generating PET images.
- PET detectors should have high stopping power, fine intrinsic spatial resolution, and good energy and timing resolution to ensure optimal PET image quality while also maintaining low readout complexity and material cost.
- The recent advancements in PET detectors include the increasing use of silicon photomultiplier technology, advances in depth-of-interaction and time-of-flight PET detectors, and the use of artificial intelligence technologies for detector development.

INTRODUCTION

PET is an in vivo imaging device that allows the assessment of various functional and biochemical processes occurring in the living bodies. In medicine, it is widely used for the diagnosis of various diseases and the assessment of therapeutic effects.[1–4] PET is also a powerful research tool that allows for a deep comprehension of the human body's function and metabolism, thereby enabling the development of innovative diagnostic and treatment approaches to various medical conditions.[5–7]

Radioactive isotopes used in PET imaging are unstable nuclides that lack neutrons and are stabilized by emitting positrons with specific half-lives. After traveling a certain distance (the positron range), the positron, which has lost most of its kinetic energy, meets the electron, leading to the mutual annihilation into 511 keV photons. PET is a tomography system that detects the annihilation photons and provides images of the spatiotemporal distribution of radiotracers labeled with the positron emitters.

To efficiently detect the annihilation photons, most PET systems use scintillation detectors consisting of inorganic scintillation crystal and photodetectors. Coincident annihilation photon pairs measured by the PET detectors within a narrow time interval (several nanoseconds) allow the lines-of-response (LORs) to be determined without mechanical collimators. This annihilation coincidence detection mechanism used in PET contributes to

[a] Department of Nuclear Medicine, Seoul National University College of Medicine, Seoul 03080, South Korea;
[b] Brightonix Imaging Inc., Seoul 04782, South Korea; [c] Environmental Radioactivity Assessment Team, Nuclear Emergency & Environmental Protection Division, Korea Atomic Energy Research Institute, Daejeon 34057, South Korea
* Corresponding author. 111, Daedeok-daero 989beon-gil, Yuseong-gu, Daejeon 34057, South Korea.
E-mail address: mslee1024@gmail.com

PET Clin 19 (2024) 1–24
https://doi.org/10.1016/j.cpet.2023.06.003

its significantly higher sensitivity compared with single-photon emission computed tomography.

There are various physical and technical factors that determine PET image quality but the most critical one is PET detector technology. PET detectors provide the essential information necessary for generating PET images, including the number of detected annihilation photons and associate physical quantities like time and energy. Therefore, in this review, the desired properties of PET detectors, including high stopping power, spatial resolution, energy resolution, and timing resolution, will be discussed (**Fig. 1** and **Table 1**). Furthermore, the recent advancements in PET detectors to improve these properties will be reviewed. These major advancements include the increasing use of silicon photomultiplier (SiPM) technology, advances in depth-of-interaction (DOI) and time-of-flight (TOF) PET detectors, and the use of artificial intelligence (AI) technologies for detector development.

DESIRED PROPERTIES OF POSITRON EMISSION TOMOGRAPHY DETECTORS
High Stopping Power Scintillator

The noise level of a PET image is mainly determined by the number of annihilation photon pairs collected by PET detectors, which can be increased by the improved stopping power of the scintillation crystal. This is because counting statistics of the scintillation detector follows a Poisson distribution. Complete stopping of high-energy (511 keV) annihilation photons is particularly important in PET because valid LORs are obtained only when both annihilation photons are detected by photoelectric absorption. Using scintillation crystal with high stopping power is also crucial in reducing intercrystal scattering (ICS) events, which reduces errors in determining the LORs, ultimately, improving the quality of PET

images.[8,9] The higher stopping power of scintillation crystal also improves the spatial resolution of PET system by mitigating parallax errors caused by obliquely incident annihilation photons penetrating the scintillation crystal.[10]

Fine Intrinsic Spatial Resolution

High spatial resolution in PET imaging is critical for accurate lesion detection, staging, and treatment response monitoring. The spatial resolution of the PET image is determined by several factors, including the intrinsic spatial resolution of PET detector, the positron range of positron emitter, the diameter of PET detector ring, parallax error, and the image reconstruction algorithm.[11,12] As the PET ring diameter decreases, the reconstructed spatial resolution improves due to the reduced effect of annihilation photon pair's noncollinearity. Therefore, small-animal and organ-dedicated PET scanners require the PET detectors with better intrinsic spatial resolution than clinical whole-body PET scanners. The intrinsic spatial resolution of the PET detector is determined by several factors, including the width of scintillation crystal elements, the ratio between crystal width and length, the pixel size of photosensors, the thickness of light guide, and the signal multiplexing method.

Fine Energy Resolution

In 3D PET systems without interplane septa, up to 50% of the events measured by the PET detector are Compton scatter events.[13] In addition, the ratio of intrascintillation scattering events is substantial in high-resolution PET detectors composed of narrow scintillation crystal elements.[14] In order to effectively remove these Compton scattering events using energy information, a PET detector must have precise energy resolution. Compton scattering correction methods based on Monte Carlo or analytical simulations[15–17] and various

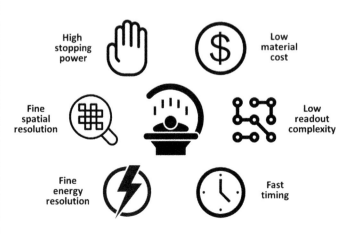

Fig. 1. Desired properties of PET detectors.

Table 1
Desired properties of scintillation crystal and photosensor to improve positron emission tomography detectors

	Scintillation Crystal	Photosensor
Stopping power	• High density and effective atomic number • Long (thick) scintillation crystal	
Spatial resolution	• Small scintillator cross section	• High photon detection efficiency (PDE)
Energy resolution	• Low intrinsic energy resolution • High photon yield	• High PDE
Timing resolution	• Fast scintillator (short rising and decay time) • High photon yield	• Low impedance • High PDE • Good single photon time resolution
Readout complexity	• Pixelated crystal array	• Large element size
Material cost	• Low raw material cost • Low melting temperature	• Semiconductor

methods for finding the first interaction position of ICS event[14,18–20] also require precise energy information. The energy resolution, which is the ability to determine the energy of incident gamma ray, of a scintillation detector is determined by the quality of the electrical signal finally produced by the detector. Therefore, the number of visible and ultraviolet photons generated in the scintillation crystal in proportion to the annihilation photon energy should be large and consistent. The light collection and quantum efficiencies of the photosensor should be high, and the amount of electrical noise generated by the intrinsic properties of the photosensor (eg, thermal noise, optical cross talk, and so forth) should be low. Proper noise management (reduction and suppression) of accompanying electronics is also essential.

Fast Timing

The coincidence measurement of PET requires a high level of precision in the timing measurement of the PET detectors. The timing resolution of a PET detector refers to the level of precision with which it can measure the differences between the arrival times of 2 annihilation photons (TOF) produced by a positron emitter. As the timing resolution of PET detectors and systems improves, the quality of PET images is enhanced, reducing the scan time and radiation dose and improving the reliability of PET scan readings.[21–23] The noise reduction also leads to the improved lesion detectability by enabling the utilization of small pixels. In addition, the TOF information is useful for overcoming the missing and inconsistent data, allowing the more accurate PET image reconstruction with limited angular samples and mitigating errors due to inconsistent correction data required for quantitative PET image generation.[24–26] TOF information also contributes to increasing the accuracy of simultaneous emission and transmission image reconstruction[27,28] and enables transmission scans using the intrinsic radioactivity of lutetium oxide crystals,[29] accelerating advances in computed tomography (CT)-less PET attenuation correction technology.[30,31] Additionally, a pair of PET detectors that measure TOF with perfect accuracy can pinpoint the origins of annihilation photons, allowing tomographic images to be generated without traditional backprojection-based image reconstruction.[32,33]

In the PET systems, coincidence logic input is generated by applying trigger electronics such as leading-edge discriminator (LED) or constant-fraction discriminator (CFD) to the rising edge of the scintillation pulse (analog output electronic signal from photosensor). The primary contributors to timing uncertainty in TOF information measurement are time walk and jitter in this trigger mechanism, which result from variations in the triggering time caused by differences and noise in the amplitude of input signal. Therefore, the PET detector and electronics should be designed to minimize them. A low slope and a high noise level of the rising edge of the scintillation pulse increase the time walk and jitter, respectively. Therefore, fast scintillator, photosensor, and electronics reduce time walk, whereas bright scintillator, efficient photosensor, low-noise electronics reduce time jitter improve the timing resolution of PET detectors.

Because the 3D PET system does not use a mechanical collimator and interplane septa, the number of high-energy photons entering PET detectors is significantly higher than that of a gamma camera, indicating that the dead time of the PET detector should be also minimized. Therefore, short decay time of scintillation crystal is also preferred.

Low Readout Complexity

With the replacement of photomultiplier tubes (PMTs) by semiconductor photosensors, the number of photosensors per scintillation crystal elements in PET detectors increases. Consequently, the increased number of output channels from the photosensors places a higher load on the subsequent data acquisition system. Therefore, various commercial or research application-specific integrated circuit chips have been developed and used to handle the high volume of signals. Moreover, numerous analog signal multiplexing techniques have been proposed to reduce the number of output channels coming from PET detectors.[34–40] However, the use of analog multiplexing may elevate the signal noise level and dispersion, consequently lowering the detector performance. Therefore, special efforts should be made to minimize the negative impact of signal multiplexing.[40] To enable flexible detector configurations and easy scalability of the system, PET detectors should be designed to be compact and modular.

Low Material Cost

PET detectors should be affordable to enable more widespread use of PET imaging in clinical and research settings. Scintillation crystals and photosensors account for a significant portion of the material cost of the PET system. The cost of photosensors is expected to decrease with the increased use of semiconductor technology. However, the price of lutetium oxide crystals (Lutetium Oxy-Orthosilicate [LSO], Lutetium-Yttrium Oxy-Orthosilicate [LYSO], and Lutetium-Gadolinium Oxy-Orthosilicate [LGSO]) currently used in high-performance PET systems continues to increase. To address this challenge, it is necessary to develop more economical scintillators that can replace lutetium oxide crystals without compromising the performance of PET systems. Alternatively, new economical approaches for detecting annihilation photons need to be explored.

RECENT ADVANCES IN POSITRON EMISSION TOMOGRAPHY DETECTOR TECHNOLOGY
Silicon Photomultiplier

PMTs have long been a major component of indirect radiation detectors because they have high-detection efficiency for visible light generated from scintillation crystals and are robust to external environmental changes such as temperature and humidity. However, PMT, which has been with PET since its birth, is being rapidly replaced as digital PET is becoming mainstream with the emergence and advances in SiPM technology (**Fig. 2**). The development of a PET system using an avalanche photodiode (APD) introduced in the 1970s was particularly active in the PET/MRI field.[41–43] However, because the internal gain of the electrical signal amplification of the APD was as low as 1/1000 of the photomultiplier tube, the PET detector based on it did not provide satisfactory performance. In the 1980s, the single-photon avalanche diode (SPAD) was proposed to detect individual photons with high signal amplification gain, similar to that of PMT. However, the SPAD, which operates in Geiger mode, was found to be unsuitable for use in PET detectors. This is because PET detectors should estimate the energy of annihilation photons by measuring the intensity of the scintillation light, whereas the output signal of the SPAD remains constant regardless of the amount of light that enters it. Developed in the 1990s, SiPM solved this problem by connecting an SPAD array in parallel. The electrical signals generated by the thousands of SPADs that are activated by the incoming photons are summed together, resulting in the SiPM's output signal that is proportional to the number of scintillation photons detected and allowing for the energy measurement of annihilation photons.[44–46]

The SiPM has subsequently attracted the attention of the PET community due to its ability of photon counting and its other desirable properties, such as high PDE and gain, fast timing, low supply voltage, compact size, and MRI compatibility.[49–51] The basic properties of SiPMs coupled with lutetium oxide crystals were investigated,[52,53] and MRI compatibility of SiPM-based scintillation detectors was tested.[54,55] The first prototype PET scanners developed using SiPM-based PET detectors showed great potential of this breakthrough technology.[56,57] Furthermore, several research groups have successfully developed MRI-compatible SiPM PET inserts,[58–63] enabling simultaneous PET/MR imaging and leading to the commercialization of SiPM-based preclinical and clinical PET/MRI solutions.[64–67] Finally, the digital PET/CT era has begun, with significantly improved detector and system performance compared with conventional PMT-based analog PET/CT.[68–70] The compactness of SiPMs mentioned previously helps to reduce scintillation light loss and enhances crystal resolving power, thereby improving the spatial, timing, and energy resolution of PET

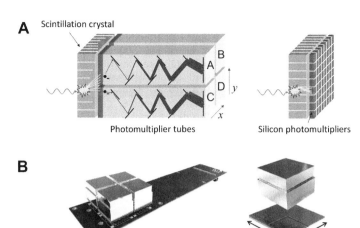

A

Scintillation crystal

Photomultiplier tubes

Silicon photomultipliers

B

26 mm

26 mm

Fig. 2. SiPM PET detectors: (*A*) Comparison between PMT and SiPM PET detectors. (*B*) Compact PET detectors based on array type SiPMs. (*From*[47,48]; with permission.)

detectors and the quality of reconstructed images. Additionally, replacing PMTs with SiPMs has reduced material costs, making it possible to develop long-axial field-of-view PET systems that allow for half-body or total-body imaging in a single bed position.[71,72]

Advancements in SiPM technology hold promise for improving PET detector and system performance. SiPMs have undergone significant development to improve their PDE and minimize unwanted noise caused by dark noise, optical cross talk, and after-pulses.[75] Moreover, the spectral range of SiPMs is being extended to cover wider wavelengths of photons,[73] enabling detection of signals in the ultraviolet region critical for detecting Cherenkov photons, which enables fast timing measurement in PET, and matching the emission wavelength of various crystals[73,76] (**Fig. 3A**). Recent research is also focused on improving the timing resolution of SiPMs by minimizing noise and quenching capacity, mitigating border effects, and optimizing single photon time resolution and pulse postprocessing.[77] Another area of development is 3D digital SiPM technology to overcome the tradeoff between PDE and performance in 2D SiPMs, in which electronic circuit limits the active area for photon detection.[74,78] In 3D digital SiPMs, each photodiode is connected to analog and digital readout electronics that are stacked on top of it, reducing dead space and enhancing PDE (**Fig. 3B**). This technology can fully use state-of-the-art electronics technology that is tailored to specific applications, resulting in improved performance.[74]

Depth-of-Interaction Detectors

As described above, the spatial resolution of the PET system can be improved by reducing the

diameter of the PET system or by using scintillation crystal elements with small frontal surface size (cross-sectional size). However, in order to maintain high PET sensitivity, it is desirable not to reduce the length of the scintillator as much as possible. The low aspect ratio (crystal cross-sectional size/crystal length) of scintillation crystal elements in the high-resolution PET systems results in the degradation of radial spatial resolution at the peripheral transverse field-of-view of PET scanner due to parallax error. The parallax error is also significant in the axial direction of 3D PET systems due to the large amount of oblique LOR accepted. The DOI measurement techniques, which measure the interaction depth of annihilation photons within the scintillation crystal, are useful for preventing the degradation of spatial resolution uniformity in PET images caused by parallax error. This DOI information can also be used to correct the DOI-dependent time-walk of the scintillation photons, helping to improve the time resolution of the PET detectors.[79]

Therefore, various innovative methods have been developed to measure the DOI position in scintillation crystals.[79] One of the most comprehensively investigated methods is to estimate the DOI position by measuring the light outputs at both ends of a pixelated crystal array (dual-ended readout) and comparing them.[80–82] When applied to an unpolished or lightly polished crystal arrays, this method provides highly accurate and precise DOI information based on a ratio of light output having a linear relationship with the DOI position. It has been also shown that the accurate DOI information obtained through the dual-ended DOI method is useful for improving TOF measurements. SiPMs enable the compact design of dual-ended DOI detectors and allow for the investigation on the feasibility of various uncommon

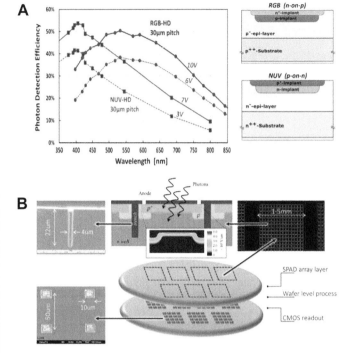

Fig. 3. Advancement in SiPM technology: (*A*) Extended spectral range: PDE of ultraviolet-sensitive SiPM (near-ultraviolet high density [NUV-HD]) compared with visible light-sensitive SiPM (RGB-HD). (*B*) 3D digital SiPM architecture. (*From*[73], Parent S, Côté M, Vachon F, Groulx R, Martel S, Dautet H, et al. Single photon avalanche diodes and vertical integration process for a 3D digital SiPM using industrial semiconductor technologies. Proc IEEE Nucl Sci Symp Med Imaging Conf 2018;1:1-4. with permission.)

arrangements of photosensors to improve the cost-effectiveness of this approach[83–85] (**Fig. 4**).

DOI estimation relying solely on the light output measurement at a single side of a scintillation crystal (single-ended readout) can reduce the cost of photosensors required for DOI measurement, compared with dual-ended readout. The most common approaches to single-ended readout include relative-offset and pulse-shape analysis methods and combination thereof.[86] The relative-offset methods involve stacking crystal arrays with half-crystal offset in either the horizontal or vertical direction (or both) to estimate both the 2D photon interaction coordinates (*x*, *y*), and the DOI position in the detector's 2D flood map.[87–89] The relatively ease of implementing relative-offset methods has led to the development of numerous clinical and preclinical PET systems using this approach.[90–92] Tailoring the scintillation light distribution by using unique arrangements of light reflectors also allow for DOI estimation from the flood map without using relative-offset of crystals[93–95] (**Fig. 5**). The light-tailoring methods implemented using only a single layer of scintillation crystal array can overcome the disadvantages of the relative-offset methods, such as errors caused by imperfect coupling and offsets between crystal layers.

Pulse-shape analysis methods offer an alternative approach to DOI estimation using single-ended readout, which can be implemented using crystal arrays with different decay times or coated with wavelength shifters.[96–99] There was also work related to DOI estimation using changes in signal rise time of either a single long crystal or 2 layers of the same crystal type.[100,101] The advantage of the rise time work is that it uses the same crystal type, and so in principle, timing resolution is not compromised. Compared with the relative-offset method, pulse-shape analysis can more easily resolve scintillation crystal positions in flood maps due to fewer crystal peaks. However, high-frequency sampling analog-to-digital converters (ADCs) are required to obtain a sufficient number of data samples for pulse-shape-based DOI estimation. To address this challenge, waveform digitization methods that do not require high-frequency sampling ADCs and pulse-shape discrimination methods that use time-over-threshold approaches have been proposed,[102,103] offering potential solutions to reduce the complexity of implementing pulse-shape analysis methods.

The degree of scintillation light dispersion is an important source of DOI information. A deeper DOI position (closer to the photosensor) leads to a narrower light distribution, which is measured by photosensor array. Measuring the degree of light dispersion or its surrogate (eg, peak to average ratio) is a commonly used method to estimate DOI in a monolithic crystal slab,[104] which has been further enhanced by using SiPM arrays with high quantum efficiency and packing fraction.

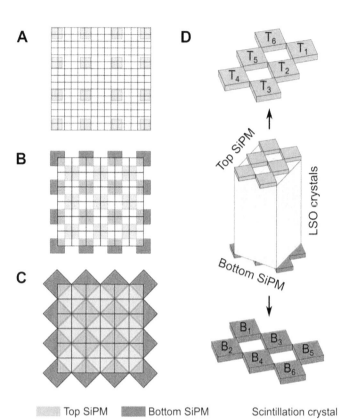

Fig. 4. Cost-effective design of dual-ended DOI detectors base on a sparse SiPM arrangement: (*A*) Dual-sided position-sensitive sparse-sensor detector (Top SiPM and Bottom SiPM are overlapped in the same position).[85] (*B*) Dichotomous offset quadrant-sharing detector design.[83] (*C, D*) 2D and 3D drawings of 45° tilted SiPMs.[84] (*From*[84]; with permission.)

Top SiPM   Bottom SiPM   Scintillation crystal

The advantages of monolithic crystal-based PET detectors include complete crystal pack fraction within a detector module and reduced crystal manufacturing costs compared with pixelated crystals.[105] However, restricted light spread at the edge of the crystal slab results in event positioning distortion. This challenge is exacerbated by increasing crystal slab thickness, which is in trade-off relationship with annihilation photon detection sensitivity. Additionally, scintillation light spread across numerous photosensors restricts timing performance. To address these issues, quasi-monolithic or semi-monolithic crystal-based detector designs have been proposed and investigated.[106–108] In these designs, multiple thin crystal slabs are stacked in the x-direction, whereas (y, z) coordinates are determined by light spread along the y-axis. This approach, which lies between pixelated and monolithic crystal-based detectors, has the potential to improve temporal resolution by increasing the number of photons collected by each photosensor.[108]

Utilization of pixelated crystals with partial optical isolation also enables DOI encoding into light dispersion, while addressing the limitations of monolithic crystals but increasing manufacturing costs. Triangular optical reflectors placed between pixelated crystals allows for the light spread-based

DOI encoding[109,110] (**Fig. 6**). By coupling a pair of pixelated crystals with respective photosensors and partially isolating them using triangular reflectors, events detected at the proximal position to the upper vertex of the triangle make the distribution of detected light more uniform.[109] Tailoring 2D DOI-dependent light dispersion in the crystal array is also possible by using and crossing the reflector strips with triangular teeth.[110,111] This approach encodes DOI information into both the direction and degree of light spread, allowing better DOI resolution to be obtained for thick crystals. Optical transparency at the top of the pixelated crystal array is achievable by using rectangular reflectors shorter than the crystal thickness or by covering the crystal array with a thin flat optical guide (**Fig. 7**).[112,113] The use of segmented prismatoid light-guide array instead of a flat optical guide has been also proposed to enhance the inter-crystal light-sharing ratios by confining light sharing to crystals coupled to the same prismatoid, thus improving crystal identification and DOI resolution.[114]

Although DOI resolution is obviously important, some of the DOI estimation methods come at the expense of degraded timing resolution or practicality of implementation. Therefore, the pros and cons of the various DOI estimation methods

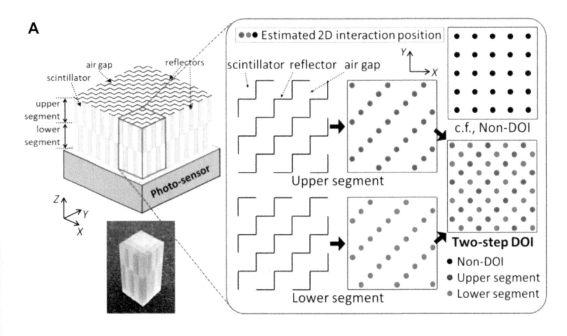

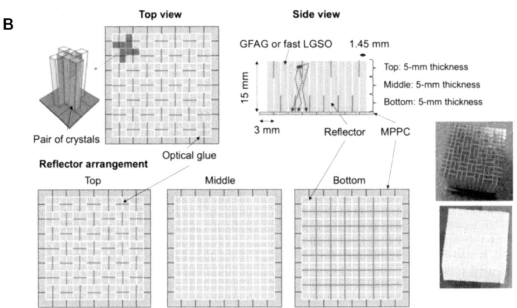

Fig. 5. DOI encoding by tailoring the scintillation light distribution by using unique arrangements of light reflectors: (*A*) Stair-shaped reflector arrangement. (*B*) Crosshair light sharing. (*From*[94,95]; with permission.)

reviewed in this article are summarized in **Table 2** to help readers' choice.

Fast Timing

The advent of LSO crystals and its derivatives, namely LYSO and LGSO, marked a major breakthrough in clinical PET systems, owing to their remarkable properties, such as short rise and decay time, high stopping power, and light output. These features offer improved timing resolution and reconstructed image quality, which are essential for clinical applications. Nevertheless, the lack of notable alternatives to cerium-doped lutetium oxide crystals remains a major hurdle. However, it has been demonstrated that the timing properties of lutetium oxide crystals can be enhanced by introducing codopants, including Ca and Mn (**Fig. 8**).[115–117]

The use of long and narrow scintillation crystal in a PET detector can result in a loss of scintillation

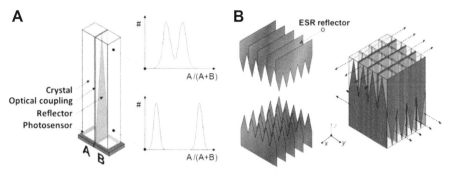

Fig. 6. DOI encoding using triangular optical reflectors: (*A*) Partial isolation of a pair of pixelated crystals using triangular reflector. (*B*) Crossing the reflector strips with triangular teeth. (*From*[9,111]; with permission.)

light because significant number of photons may not be able to enter the photosensor due to small solid angle. Inorganic scintillation crystals, which typically have a high refractive index, may also experience total internal reflection at the scintillation crystal and photosensor boundary, leading to further scintillation light loss. Consequently, ongoing research aims to optimize light extraction from scintillation crystals by applying an optimized surface treatment and using appropriate reflective materials, such as diffusive or specular reflectors, to improve light collection efficiency. Furthermore, dual-ended readout is more effective than single-ended readout in terms of both light collection and timing resolution.[118,119] With the advent of thin SiPM technology, side-readout has become a more feasible option, offering further improvements in light collection (**Fig. 9**).[120–122] To achieve higher light-collection efficiency, SiPMs with high PDE that better match with scintillation photon wavelength should be used.

To overcome the total internal reflection issue, the use of photonic crystals has been also proposed. Photonic crystals consist of a thin slab with a regular array of nanoholes that scatter the light in multiple directions and enhance the probability of light extraction[123] (**Fig. 10**). Another noticeable nanotechnology for improving the timing

performance of PET detectors is the nanocrystals with high quantum efficiency and ultrafast timing properties, such as CdSe and $CsPbBr_3$ nanoplatelets.[124,125] These nanocrystals are ultrafast emitting quantum confined systems with sub-100 picoseconds decay time and can potentially be combined with heavy inorganic scintillators, such as LSO and BGO, to form a metascintillator, which will be further described later in this review.[33]

BGO replaced NaI(Tl) in the early days of PET development and was widely used as a scintillator for PET scanners. However, with the introduction of LSO, its use has declined significantly. Nonetheless, BGO is once again attracting attention due to the ultrafast Cherenkov light photons generated on detection of 511 keV annihilation photons.[126,127] The emission of scintillation photons is a slow process, elapsed over 10^{-8} seconds after the electron leaves the orbit by photoelectric absorption or Compton scattering, whereas Cherenkov photons are emitted almost instantaneously when electrons move with the highest kinetic energy and speed faster than that of light in the scintillation crystal. Recently, 32 ps timing resolution could be achieved by using a combination of pure Cherenkov emitter (lead glass), microchannel plates PMT, and deep learning based timing measurement, enabling the generation of positron

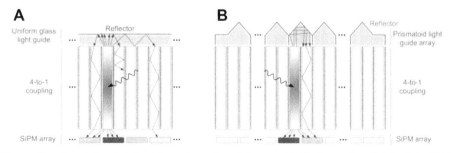

Fig. 7. DOI encoding by adding light guide on top of crystal array: (*A*) Uniform glass light guide. (*B*) Prismatoid light guide. (This research was originally published in JNM. LaBella A, Cao X, Petersen E, Lubinsky R, Biegon A, Zhao W, et al. High-resolution depth-encoding PET detector module with prismatoid light-guide array. J Nucl Med. 2020;61(10):1528-33. © SNMMI.)

Table 2
Pros and cons of various depth-of-interaction estimation methods reviewed in this article

	Pros	Cons
Dual-ended readout using dense photosensor array[80–82]	• Highly accurate DOI and timing estimation	• Increased photosensor cost and readout complexity
Dual-ended readout with sparse photosensor arrangement[83–85]	• Reduced photosensor cost and readout complexity	• Compromised DOI and timing resolution
Relative-offset methods with half-crystal offset[87–89]	• DOI estimation from flood maps • Relatively easy implementation	• Dense population of crystal peaks in flood map • Errors caused by inaccurate offsets between crystal layers
Pseudo relative-offset methods with nontraditional reflector arrangement[93–95]	• DOI estimation from flood maps • Reduction of errors caused by inaccurate offsets	• Dense population of crystal peaks in flood map • Increased complexity in crystal array assembly
Pulse-shape analysis on different decay time[96–99]	• Fewer crystal peaks in flood maps compared with relative-offset methods	• Increased readout complexity for pulse-shape analysis • Increased detector deadtime and compromised timing resolution
Pulse-shape analysis on different rise time[100,101]	• Fewer crystal peaks • No timing resolution compromise	• Increased readout complexity for pulse-shape analysis
Light-dispersion analysis with fully monolithic crystal[104,105]	• Reduced crystal cost • Complete crystal packing fraction	• Increased readout complexity for light-dispersion analysis • Positing distortion at crystal edge • Compromised timing resolution
Light-dispersion analysis with semi-monolithic crystal[106–108]	• Modest crystal cost • Improved positioning accuracy and timing performance	• Increased readout complexity for light-dispersion analysis
Light-dispersion analysis with pixelated crystal[109–114]	• Highly accurate 3D positing accuracy through single-ended readout and single-type crystal	• Increased readout complexity for light-dispersion analysis

emission images without the need for conventional backprojection-based image reconstruction methods (**Fig. 11**).[32] The amount of Cherenkov photons produced is inversely related to the speed of light in a medium, and materials with higher refractive indices produce more Cherenkov radiation. Researchers are thus exploring Cherenkov radiators with high refractive indices, such as TlBr, TlCr, $CsPbCl_3$, and $CsPbBr_3$.[128,129] As the wavelength decreases, the amount of Cherenkov radiation produced increases. Because each crystal has a different cut-off wavelength, it is important to select a SiPM with an appropriate spectral range (eg, $PbF2$: 250 nm, BGO: 300 nm, TlCl: 400 nm, TlBr: 440 nm).[129] The measurement of Cherenkov radiation has the potential to enhance timing resolution of PET. However, due

to the relatively low amount of Cherenkov photons produced, the sensitivity of annihilation photon detection is reduced, and energy estimation becomes challenging. To overcome these obstacles, the use of a crystal that emits both scintillation and Cherenkov radiation is advantageous compared with a pure Cherenkov radiator. Such a crystal can provide improved sensitivity for detecting annihilation photons and allow more accurate energy estimation.

BGO has garnered considerable interest from the scientific community owing to its affordability, as well as its property of emitting both Cherenkov and scintillation photons (**Fig. 12**). BGO's high refractive index makes it favorable material for generating Cherenkov photons, although they are relatively few in number (17 photons for a 511 keV

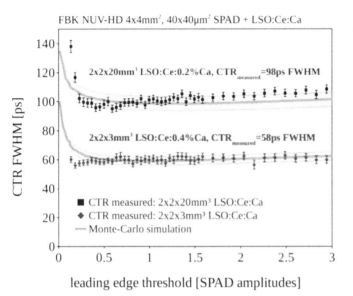

FBK NUV-HD 4x4mm², 40x40µm² SPAD + LSO:Ce:Ca

2x2x20mm³ LSO:Ce:0.2%Ca, CTR$_{measured}$=98ps FWHM

2x2x3mm³ LSO:Ce:0.4%Ca, CTR$_{measured}$=58ps FWHM

■ CTR measured: 2x2x20mm³ LSO:Ce:Ca
◆ CTR measured: 2x2x3mm³ LSO:Ce:Ca
— Monte-Carlo simulation

leading edge threshold [SPAD amplitudes]

Fig. 8. Timing resolution of LSO:Ce co-doped with Ca. (From[115]; with permission.)

event) and are primarily in the ultraviolet range. By using $3 \times 3 \times 15$ mm³ BGO crystals and NUV-HD SiPMs, a timing resolution of better than 300 picoseconds FWHM (full-width at half-maximum) was achieved.[115,130] Nevertheless, the use of broadband RF amplifiers for SiPM signal readout electronics in these experiments posed challenges due to their high power consumption and sensitivity to noise. To facilitate system-level upscaling, it is essential to conduct further research on readout electronics that are cost-effective, power-efficient, compact, and robust.[131] Moreover, it is worth noting that the timing performance of BGO cannot be fully represented by a single FWHM value because its timing distribution has a long tail. This is because events triggered from BGO detectors are a combination of Cherenkov and scintillation events, which results in different timing resolutions depending on the type of event that triggers the signal. Event-by-event classification of Cherenkov and scintillation events has the potential to enhance the quality of reconstructed images because using proper timing kernel is important for TOF PET image reconstruction.[132,133] Finally, to enhance the generation of Cherenkov light and improve the efficiency of light collection, comprehensive research on new

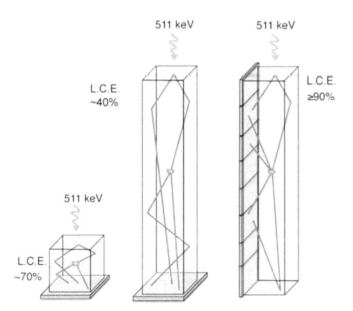

511 keV   511 keV

L.C.E. ~40%

L.C.E. ≥90%

511 keV

L.C.E. ~70%

Fig. 9. Improved light-collection efficiency (L.C.E.) by side-readout of crystal. (From[120]; with permission.)

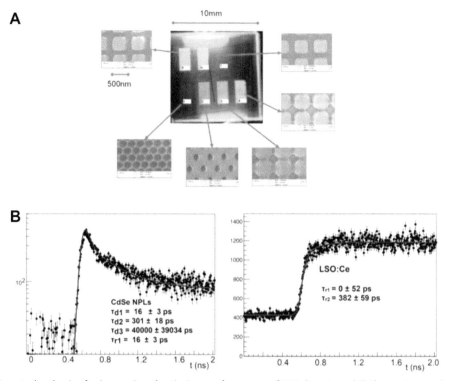

Fig. 10. Nanotechnologies for improving the timing performance of PET detectors: (*A*) Photonic crystal. (*B*) Nanocrystals: luminescence response of the CdSe nanoplatelets deposited on top of LSO (left) and conventional LSO (right) in the first 2 ns. (*From*[123,124]; with permission.)

materials, sensors, and light readout techniques is also necessary.

Metascintillator is another relatively new technique proposed to overcome the slow development of fast inorganic scintillators with sufficiently high stopping power for 511 keV annihilation photons.[134] Compared with other emerging technologies, metascintillators seem to be relatively close to practical use. Metascintillators consist of alternating thin slabs (100–300 μm) of heavy, dense inorganic scintillation crystals, such as LSO and BGO, and light but fast plastic scintillators or BaF$_2$ that emits fast cross-luminescence (**Fig. 13**).[135,136] When photoelectric recoil electrons are ejected mainly from the heavy inorganic scintillator, they travel across the alternating thin slabs, enabling the emission of fast photons. Consequently, combining fast materials with lutetium oxide crystals and BGO-based PET detectors can improve timing resolution at the cost of detection efficiency. Using 3 × 3 × 15 mm^3 BGO and EJ232 (plastic scintillator) metascintillator, coincidence timing resolutions (CTRs) of 239 picoseconds and 197 picoseconds were obtained with 100-μm and 200-μm thick EJ232 slabs, respectively (both in combination with 100-μm thick BGO plates). These values represent a significant

improvement over the 271-picosecond and 303-picosecond CTRs with bulk and layered BGO, respectively.[137] Moreover, a 3 × 3 × 15 mm^3 metascintillator consisting of 300 μm BGO and 300 μm BaF$_2$ layers yielded a CTR of 241 picoseconds while maintaining radiation stopping power equivalent to LSO.[138]

In the past, techniques for measuring TOF information in small ring PET systems, such as brain-dedicated or breast-dedicated PET scanners, have not received much attention because the time resolution of PET detectors was not sufficiently good for improving the image quality of these small ring PET systems. However, with fine time resolution of PET detectors in 100-picosecond level that provides LOR constraints of 1.5 cm in the image reconstruction process, small ring PET systems can also benefit from TOF capability, resulting in enhanced image SNR. Hence, the importance of detector technology that can accurately measure both DOI and TOF information has increased.[121] Achieving a DOI resolution that is comparable to the intrinsic spatial resolution of PET detectors would be sufficient to attain uniform spatial resolution across the field-of-view. Consequently, enhancing the timing resolution should be the primary focus if the DOI resolution of a PET

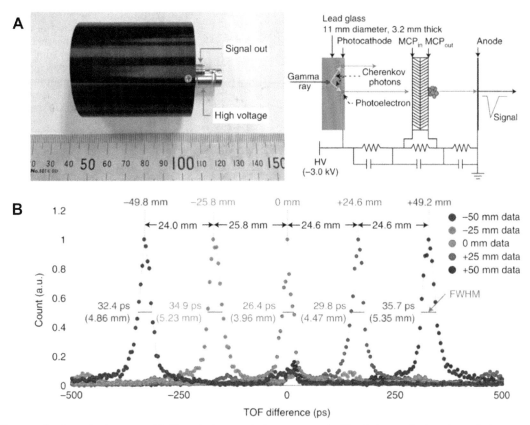

Fig. 11. Ultrafast PET detector with 32 ps timing resolution composed of lead glass and microchannel plates PMT: (A) Detector configuration. (B) Timing histogram. (From[32]; with permission.)

detector has already attained the level of its intrinsic spatial resolution.

Artificial Intelligence

After AlphaGo defeated Go master Lee Se-dol in 2016, machine learning and AI technology attracted explosive attention from scientists and engineers around the world and took a huge leap to an unreachable level before. AI technology has become the main mainstream in almost all areas of biomedical image processing and interpretation research.[139–142] In various fields of PET image generation, AI technology is outperforming conventional mathematical algorithms. In addition, AI technology is contributing to the development of PET imaging technology by improving the performance of existing image correction and reconstruction algorithms or by supplementing their shortcomings.[30,143–145] Currently, these AI technologies are not limited to the field of PET image processing but are being used in various attempts to improve the performance of PET detectors and readout technologies and enhance their functions.[146,147] For example, neural networks have

emerged as a popular technique for accurately determining the 3D positioning of photon interactions within monolithic crystals (**Fig. 14**).[105,148–150] Here are additional examples of recent attempts to leverage AI technologies on the PET hardware side.

The timing resolution of PET detectors can be improved using fast waveform digitizers and deep neural networks. The time-elapsing scintillation process and limited time response of photosensors and readout electronics result in a slow build-up of the scintillation pulse, which is susceptible to noise contamination. Single-threshold trigger electronics are prone to significant timing uncertainty arising from the time walk and jitter effects, as previously discussed. Multiple data points sampled at the rising edge of the scintillation pulse using fast wave digitizers, such as high-frequency free running ADCs and domino-ring samplers, provide additional information that may be useful for mitigating timing uncertainty in PET. Furthermore, artificial neural networks are effective regressors that can adequately handle noisy data with training using large datasets. For example, a convolutional neural network (CNN)

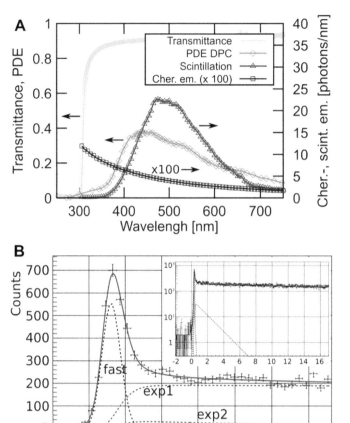

Fig. 12. Ultrafast Cherenkov photons emitted from BGO: (*A*) Spectral properties of scintillation and Cherenkov photons coming from BGO. (*B*) Luminescent response during the first 1.5 ns following excitation by 511 keV photons, illustrating a significant prompt component with 160 ps full width at half maximum (FWHM) by Cherenkov emission. (*From*[126]; with permission.)

trained with cropped rising edges of coincident pulses acquired from 5 × 5 × 10 mm³ LFS crystals coupled to single-channel PMTs as input, and their true arrival time difference calculated based on the position of a point source as the ground truth for network output, improved timing resolution by 20% compared with LED and 23% compared with CFD.[151] This approach was also useful for attaining the 32 picoseconds CTR of the pair of Cherenkov PET detectors, comprising lead glass

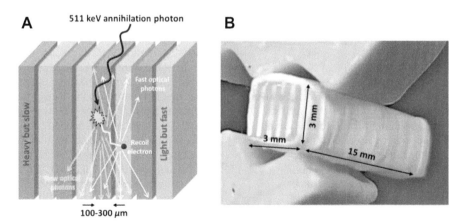

Fig. 13. Metascintillator: (*A*) Conceptual drawing of metascintillator that is alternating thin slabs of heavy, dense inorganic scintillation crystals and light but fast plastic scintillators. (*B*) BGO:BaF₂ metascintillator. (*From*[138]; with permission.)

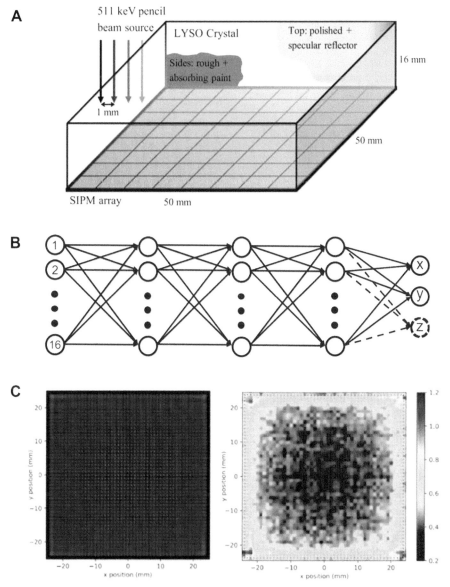

Fig. 14. Positioning of gamma-ray interactions in monolithic detectors using an artificial neural network: (*A*) Detector and experimental setup. (*B*) Neural network architecture. (*C*) Predicted positions and position error. (*From*[150]; with permission.)

and microchannel plates PMT.[32] In addition, an unbiased estimator of arrival time difference, which combines LED and CNN trained using waveforms obtained from a single source position, has been proposed.[152] Specifically, a CNN that estimates the time difference error from the shifted and cropped rising edges of sampled waveforms improved the CTR by approximately 10% compared with the conventional LED.

In addition, AI technology has the potential to improve the estimation accuracy of the first interaction position of ICS events in PET detectors with narrow crystal elements. Using scintillator crystal elements with narrower size to achieve higher spatial resolution in PET detectors increases the proportion of ICS relative to photoelectric interaction. For example, ICS events accounts for 42% of total events in PET detector comprising a 16×16 array with $1.5 \times 1.5 \times 20 \text{ mm}^3$ LSO crystals (crystal pitch = 1.6 mm).[153] Accurate estimation of the fist interaction position of ICS events is crucial for the correct allocation of LORs. However, the identification of ICS events and the determination of the first interaction position is challenging in light-sharing detectors with crystal elements narrower than the pitch of photosensors. To

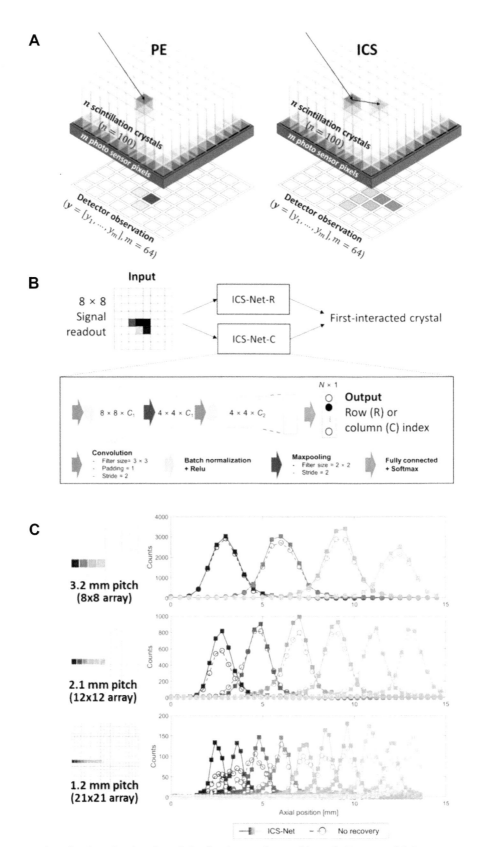

Fig. 15. Deep learning-based estimation of the first interaction position of ICS events: (*A*) Detector response for photoelectric (PE) and ICS events. (*B*) Network architecture. (*C*) Count profiles obtained with pencil beam irradiation indicating the improved intrinsic resolution. (*From*[19,154]; with permission.)

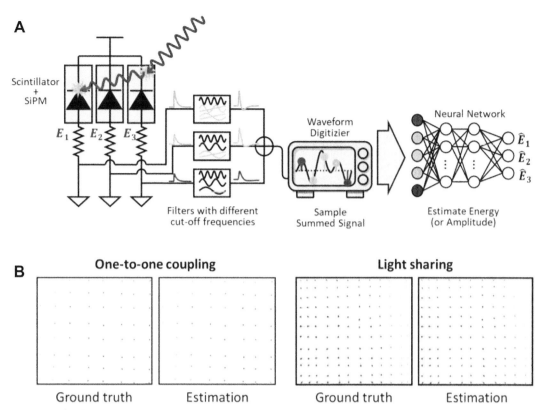

Fig. 16. Artificial neural network-based SiPM signal multiplexing: (*A*) Concept. (*B*) Experimental results: flood maps generated using the center-of-gravity algorithm applied to the true and estimated energies. (*From*[155]; with permission.)

investigate the potential usefulness of AI technology in pinpointing the first interaction positions of ICS events in light-sharing PET detectors, CNNs were trained using the 2D SiPM signal readout pattern as input and the row or column index of the first-interacted crystal (**Fig. 15**).[154] In the experimental study, the CNN-based first interaction position estimation improved the intrinsic detector resolution by 20%, 31%, and 62% for 8 × 8, 12 × 12, and 21 × 21 LSO crystal arrays with the pitches of 3.2, 2.1, and 1.2 mm, respectively, compared with conventional flood map-based crystal assignment without considering the ICS phenomenon.

AI technology can help reduce the readout complexity of PET detectors. Although SiPM's compactness offers many advantages, it also increases the number of output channels that must be handled by the subsequent readout electronics. To reduce the number of output channels from PET detectors, various signal multiplexing methods have been used. However, most of these methods use charge division networks, which calculate the centroid of output signals from photosensors. Unfortunately, these methods cannot

accurately recover the exact information on the origins and amplitude of signals when multiple photosensors yield signals simultaneously due to light sharing, ICS, and multiple coincidences. To address this challenge, an artificial neural network-based multiplexing method has been proposed.[155] In this method, the output signal from each SiPM undergoes high-pass filtering with a unique cutoff frequency, and the filtered signals are then merged into a single output signal. The artificial neural network receives the sampled waveform of the merged signal as input and infers the amplitude of each filtered signal (**Fig. 16**). The trained network with optimally designed set of filters based on the Cramér–Rao lower bound yielded an R^2 value of 0.99 between the true and estimated signals. Moreover, the 2D energy deposition distribution in the crystal array provided by this new multiplexing method was useful for identifying ICS events.

SUMMARY

PET detectors are essential components in PET imaging, and their properties significantly influence the quality of PET images. The desired properties of PET detectors include high stopping power, fine intrinsic spatial resolution, fine energy resolution, and fast timing. Scintillation crystals with high stopping power can improve the PET images quality by increasing the sensitivity of annihilation photon detection and reducing ICS events. Fine intrinsic spatial resolution, determined by the width of scintillation crystal elements, photosensor pixel size, light guide thickness, and signal multiplexing method, is critical for accurate lesion detection. Fine energy resolution is necessary for effectively removing Compton scattering events and can be achieved by using scintillation crystal with high light yield and photosensors with high light collection and quantum efficiencies. Fast timing is required to enhance PET image quality and reduce scan time and radiation dose. It can be improved by minimizing time walk and jitter through optimal design of PET detectors and electronics.

The recent advancements in PET detectors include the increasing use of SiPM technology, advances in DOI and TOF PET detectors, and the use of AI technologies for detector development. First, SiPM is replacing traditional PMTs due to their high PDE, gain, and compact size. SiPMs have also improved PET detector performance by reducing scintillation light loss and enhancing crystal resolving power, resulting in improved spatial, timing, and energy resolution. Additionally, replacing PMTs with SiPMs has reduced material costs, making it possible to develop long-axial field-of-view PET systems that allow for half-body or total-body imaging in a single bed position. Further advancements in SiPM technology are ongoing, with research focused on improving PDE, minimizing noise, and extending the spectral range to cover wider wavelengths of photons. Second, various innovative methods have been developed to measure the DOI position because the measurement of DOI of annihilation photons within the scintillation crystal is useful for improving spatial resolution uniformity and timing resolution. The degree of scintillation light dispersion is an important source of DOI information, and measuring the degree of light dispersion or its surrogate is more commonly used for estimating DOI. SiPMs enable the compact design of dual-ended DOI detectors and allow the development of novel single-ended DOI detectors with high DOI resolution. Third, active research is being conducted on various methods to improve the time resolution of PET detectors. The use of LSO crystals and their derivatives has significantly improved the timing resolution of clinical PET systems but the lack of alternatives to cerium-doped lutetium oxide crystals remains a major hurdle.

Photonic crystals to enhance the light extraction from scintillation crystals and nanocrystals with high quantum efficiency and ultrafast timing properties are also being explored to improve the timing performance of PET detectors. BGO, once widely used as a scintillator for PET scanners, is attracting attention again due to the ultrafast Cherenkov light photons generated on detection of 511 keV annihilation photons. The use of Cherenkov radiators with high refractive indices is being investigated to enhance timing resolution but the low amount of Cherenkov photons produced poses a challenge to annihilation photon detection sensitivity and energy estimation. Researchers are exploring various approaches to overcome these challenges and enhance the timing resolution of PET detectors. Finally, AI technologies are not limited to the field of PET image processing but are being used in various attempts to enhance the performance of PET detectors and readout technologies. For instance, the timing resolution of PET detectors can be improved using fast waveform digitizers and deep neural networks. AI technology also has the potential to improve the estimation accuracy of the first interaction position of ICS events in PET detectors with narrow crystal elements. Furthermore, AI technology can help reduce the readout complexity of PET detectors.

CLINICS CARE POINTS

- With advancements in PET imaging technology, we can achieve enhanced PET image quality, offering multiple clinical benefits.
- Improved PET image quality enhances the overall reliability and accuracy of PET scan readings, leading to more precise diagnostic outcomes.
- Consequently, enhanced PET image quality can reduce PET scan time with the same radiation dose, allowing higher patient turnover. Alternatively, it can reduce the radiation dose exposed to patients, prioritizing their safety and well-being.

DISCLOSURE

The authors have no relationships relevant to the contents of this paper to disclose.

ACKNOWLEDGMENTS

The authors acknowledge support by the National Research Foundation of Korea, South Korea

(Grant No. NRF-2022R1C1C1013092) and the Korea Medical Device Development Fund grant funded by the Korea government (the Ministry of Science and ICT, the Ministry of Trade, Industry and Energy, the Ministry of Health & Welfare, the Ministry of Food and Drug Safety; Project Number: 1711137868, RS-2020-KD000006). In addition, the authors thank Hyeong Seok Shim, Sangjin Bae, and Suleman Surti for their invaluable comments, which significantly improved the article.

REFERENCES

1. Marcelo FDC. Why will PET be the future of nuclear cardiology? J Nucl Med 2021;62(9):1189.
2. Raynor WY, Borja AJ, Hancin EC, et al. Novel musculoskeletal and orthopedic applications of 18F-sodium fluoride PET. Pet Clin 2021;16(2): 295–311.
3. Chavoshi M, Mirshahvalad SA, Metser U, et al. 68Ga-PSMA PET in prostate cancer: a systematic review and meta-analysis of the observer agreement. Eur J Nucl Med Mol Imaging 2022;49(3): 1021–9.
4. Dhawan V, Niethammer MH, Lesser ML, et al. Prospective F-18 FDOPA PET imaging study in human PD. Nucl Med Mol Imaging 2022;56(3):147–57.
5. Pomper MG, Lee JS. Small animal imaging in drug development. Curr Pharm Des 2005;11(25):3247–72.
6. Lamberts LE, Williams SP, Terwisscha van Scheltinga AG, et al. Antibody positron emission tomography imaging in anticancer drug development. J Clin Oncol 2015;33(13):1491–504.
7. Kang S-R, Min J-J. Recent progress in the molecular imaging of tumor-treating bacteria. Nucl Med Mol Imaging 2021;55(1):7–14.
8. Abbaszadeh S, Chinn G, Levin CS. Positioning true coincidences that undergo inter-and intra-crystal scatter for a sub-mm resolution cadmium zinc telluride-based PET system. Phys Med Biol 2018; 03(2).025012.
9. Lee S, Kim KY, Lee MS, et al. Recovery of inter-detector and inter-crystal scattering in brain PET based on LSO and GAGG crystals. Phys Med Biol 2020;65(19):195005.
10. Schmall JP, Karp JS, Werner M, et al. Parallax error in long-axial field-of-view PET scanners-a simulation study. Phys Med Biol 2016;61(14):5443–55.
11. Wang Y, Seidel J, Tsui BM, et al. Performance evaluation of the GE healthcare eXplore VISTA dual-ring small-animal PET scanner. J Nucl Med 2006; 47(11):1891–900.
12. Lecomte R. Novel detector technology for clinical PET. Eur J Nucl Med Mol Imaging 2009;36(1):69–85.
13. Thompson C. The effect of collimation on scatter fraction in multi-slice PET. IEEE Trans Nucl Sci 1988;35(1):598–602.

14. Yiping S, Cherry SR, Siegel S, et al. A study of inter-crystal scatter in small scintillator arrays designed for high resolution PET imaging. IEEE Trans Nucl Sci 1996;43(3):1938–44.
15. John MO. Model-based scatter correction for fully 3D PET. Phys Med Biol 1996;41(1):153.
16. Accorsi R, Adam LE, Werner ME, et al. Optimization of a fully 3D single scatter simulation algorithm for 3D PET. Phys Med Biol 2004;49(12): 2577–98.
17. Watson CC. New, faster, image-based scatter correction for 3D PET. IEEE Trans Nucl Sci 2000; 47(4):1587–94.
18. Comanor K, Virador P, Moses W. Algorithms to identify detector Compton scatter in PET modules. IEEE Trans Nucl Sci 1996;43(4):2213–8.
19. Lee MS, Kang SK, Lee JS. Novel inter-crystal scattering event identification method for PET detectors. Phys Med Biol 2018;63(11):115015.
20. Rafecas M, Böning G, Pichler B, et al. Inter-crystal scatter in a dual layer, high resolution LSO-APD positron emission tomograph. Phys Med Biol 2003;48(7):821–48.
21. Karp JS, Surti S, Daube-Witherspoon ME, et al. Benefit of time-of-flight in PET: experimental and clinical results. J Nucl Med 2008;49(3):462–70.
22. Vandenberghe S, Mikhaylova E, D'Hoe E, et al. Recent developments in time-of-flight PET. EJNMMI Phys 2016;3(1):3.
23. Surti S. Update on time-of-flight PET imaging. J Nucl Med 2015;56(1):98–105.
24. Surti S, Karp JS. Design considerations for a limited angle, dedicated breast, TOF PET scanner. Phys Med Biol 2008;53(11):2911–21.
25. Conti M. State of the art and challenges of time-of-flight PET. Phys Med 2009;25(1):1–11.
26. Son JW, Kim KY, Yoon HS, et al. Proof-of-concept prototype time-of-flight PET system based on high-quantum-efficiency multianode PMTs. Med Phys 2017;44(10):5314–24.
27. Defrise M, Rezaei A, Nuyts J. Time-of-flight PET data determine the attenuation sinogram up to a constant. Phys Med Biol 2012;57(4):885–99.
28. Rezaei A, Defrise M, Bal G, et al. Simultaneous reconstruction of activity and attenuation in time-of-flight PET. IEEE Trans Med Imaging 2012; 31(12):2224–33.
29. Rothfuss H, Panin V, Moor A, et al. LSO background radiation as a transmission source using time of flight. Phys Med Biol 2014;59(18): 5483–500.
30. Hwang D, Kang SK, Kim KY, et al. Generation of PET attenuation map for whole-body time-of-flight (18)F-FDG PET/MRI using a deep neural network trained with simultaneously reconstructed activity and attenuation maps. J Nucl Med 2019;60(8): 1183–9.

31. Hwang D, Kim KY, Kang SK, et al. Improving the accuracy of simultaneously reconstructed activity and attenuation maps using deep learning. J Nucl Med 2018;59(10):1624–9.

32. Kwon SI, Ota R, Berg E, et al. Ultrafast timing enables reconstruction-free positron emission imaging. Nat Photonics 2021;15(12):914–8.

33. Lecoq P, Morel C, Prior JO, et al. Roadmap toward the 10 ps time-of-flight PET challenge. Phys Med Biol 2020;65(21):21RM01.

34. Olcott PD, Glover G, Levin CS. Cross-strip multiplexed electro-optical coupled scintillation detector for integrated PET/MRI. IEEE Trans Nucl Sci 2013; 60(5):3198–204.

35. Popov V, Majewski S, Weisenberger AG. Readout electronics for multianode photomultiplier tubes with pad matrix anode layout. Proc IEEE Nucl Sci Symp Med Imaging Conf 2003;1:2156–9.

36. Siegel S, Silverman RW, Yiping S, et al. Simple charge division readouts for imaging scintillator arrays using a multi-channel PMT. IEEE Trans Nucl Sci 1996;43(3):1634–41.

37. Yoon HS, Lee JS. Bipolar analog signal multiplexing for position-sensitive PET block detectors. Phys Med Biol 2014;59(24):7835–46.

38. Won JY, Ko GB, Lee JS. Delay grid multiplexing: simple time-based multiplexing and readout method for silicon photomultipliers. Phys Med Biol 2016;61(19):7113–35.

39. Park H, Ko GB, Lee JS. Hybrid charge division multiplexing method for silicon photomultiplier based PET detectors. Phys Med Biol 2017;62(11):4390–405.

40. Park H, Yi M, Lee JS. Silicon photomultiplier signal readout and multiplexing techniques for positron emission tomography: a review. Biomed Eng Lett 2022;12(3):263–83.

41. Catana C, Procissi D, Wu Y, et al. Simultaneous in vivo positron emission tomography and magnetic resonance imaging. Proc Natl Acad Sci USA 2008;105(10):3705–10.

42. Delso G, Fürst S, Jakoby B, et al. Performance measurements of the Siemens mMR integrated whole-body PET/MR scanner. J Nucl Med 2011; 52(12):1914–22.

43. Judenhofer MS, Wehrl HF, Newport DF, et al. Simultaneous PET-MRI: a new approach for functional and morphological imaging. Nat Med 2008;14(4):459–65.

44. Bondarenko G, Buzhan P, Dolgoshein B, et al. Limited Geiger-mode microcell silicon photodiode: new results. Nucl Instrum Methods Phys Res 2000; 442(1–3):187–92.

45. Golovin V, Saveliev V. Novel type of avalanche photodetector with Geiger mode operation. Nucl Instrum Methods Phys Res 2004;518(1–2):560–4.

46. Renker D. Geiger-mode avalanche photodiodes, history, properties and problems. Nucl Instrum Methods Phys Res 2006;567(1):48–56.

47. Park H, Lee JS. Highly multiplexed SiPM signal readout for brain-dedicated TOF-DOI PET detectors. Phys Med 2019;68:117–23.

48. Won JY, Ko GB, Kim KY, et al. Comparator-less PET data acquisition system using single-ended memory interface input receivers of FPGA. Phys Med Biol 2020;65(15):155007.

49. Lee JS. Technical advances in current PET and hybrid imaging systems. Open Nucl Med J 2010; 2:192–208.

50. Lee JS, Hong SJ. Geiger-mode avalanche photodiodes for PET/MRI. In: Iniewski K, editor. Electronics for radiation detection. Boca Raton, FL: CRC Press; 2010. p. 179–99.

51. Roncali E, Cherry SR. Application of silicon photomultipliers to positron emission tomography. Ann Biomed Eng 2011;39:1358–77.

52. Otte AN, Barral J, Dolgoshein B, et al. A test of silicon photomultipliers as readout for PET. Nucl Instrum Methods Phys Res 2005;545(3):705–15.

53. Lee JS, Ito M, Sim K, et al. Investigation of solid-state photomultipliers for positron emission tomography scanners. J Korean Phys Soc 2007;50(5):1332.

54. Spanoudaki VC, Mann AB, Otte AN, et al. Use of single photon counting detector arrays in combined PET/MR: characterization of LYSO-SiPM detector modules and comparison with a LSO-APD detector. J Inst Met 2007;2(12):P12002.

55. Hong SJ, Song IC, Ito M, et al. An investigation into the Use of Geiger-mode solid-state photomultipliers for simultaneous PET and MRI acquisition. IEEE Trans Nucl Sci 2008;55(3):882–8.

56. Yamamoto S, Imaizumi M, Watabe T, et al. Development of a Si-PM-based high-resolution PET system for small animals. Phys Med Biol 2010;55(19):5817.

57. Kwon SI, Lee JS, Yoon HS, et al. Development of small-animal PET prototype using silicon photomultiplier (SiPM): initial results of phantom and animal imaging studies. J Nucl Med 2011;52(4):572–9.

58. Yoon HS, Ko GB, Kwon SI, et al. Initial results of simultaneous PET/MRI experiments with an MRI-compatible silicon photomultiplier PET scanner. J Nucl Med 2012;53(4):608–14.

59. Jung JH, Choi Y, Jung J, et al. Development of PET/MRI with insertable PET for simultaneous PET and MR imaging of human brain. Med Phys 2015; 42(5):2354–63.

60. Thiessen JD, Shams E, Stortz G, et al. MR-compatibility of a high-resolution small animal PET insert operating inside a 7 T MRI. Phys Med Biol 2016;61(22):7934–56.

61. Schug D, Lerche C, Weissler B, et al. Initial PET performance evaluation of a preclinical insert for PET/MRI with digital SiPM technology. Phys Med Biol 2016;61(7):2851.

62. Grant AM, Lee BJ, Chang CM, et al. Simultaneous PET/MR imaging with a radio frequency-penetrable PET insert. Med Phys 2017;44(1):112–20.

63. Ko GB, Yoon HS, Kim KY, et al. Simultaneous multi-parametric PET/MRI with silicon photomultiplier PET and ultra-high-field MRI for small-animal imaging. J Nucl Med 2016;57(8):1309–15.

64. Levin CS, Maramraju SH, Khalighi MM, et al. Design features and mutual compatibility studies of the time-of-flight PET capable GE SIGNA PET/MR system. IEEE Trans Med Imaging 2016;35(8):1907–14.

65. Son J-W, Kim KY, Park JY, et al. SimPET: a preclinical PET insert for simultaneous PET/MR imaging. Mol Imaging Biol 2020;22:1208–17.

66. Gsell W, Molinos C, Correcher C, et al. Characterization of a preclinical PET insert in a 7 tesla MRI scanner: beyond NEMA testing. Phys Med Biol 2020;65(24):245016.

67. Courteau A, McGrath J, Walker PM, et al. Performance evaluation and compatibility studies of a compact preclinical scanner for simultaneous PET/MR imaging at 7 Tesla. IEEE Trans Med Imaging 2021;40(1):205–17.

68. Rausch I, Ruiz A, Valverde-Pascual I, et al. Performance evaluation of the Vereos PET/CT system according to the NEMA NU2-2012 standard. J Nucl Med 2019;60(4):561–7.

69. Pan T, Einstein SA, Kappadath SC, et al. Performance evaluation of the 5-Ring GE Discovery MI PET/CT system using the national electrical manufacturers association NU 2-2012 Standard. Med Phys 2019;46(7):3025–33.

70. Carlier T, Ferrer L, Conti M, et al. From a PMT-based to a SiPM-based PET system: a study to define matched acquisition/reconstruction parameters and NEMA performance of the Biograph Vision 450. EJNMMI Phys 2020;7(1):55.

71. Cherry SR, Badawi RD, Karp JS, et al. Total-body imaging: Transforming the role of positron emission tomography. Sci Transl Med 2017;9(381):eaaf6169.

72. Prenosil GA, Sari H, Fürstner M, et al. Performance characteristics of the Biograph Vision Quadra PET/CT system with a long axial field of view using the NEMA NU 2 2018 standard. J Nucl Med 2022;63(3):476–84.

73. Acerbi F, Paternoster G, Capasso M, et al. Silicon photomultipliers: technology optimizations for ultraviolet, visible and near-infrared range. Instruments 2019;3(1):15.

74. Parent S, Côté M, Vachon F, et al. Single photon avalanche diodes and vertical integration process for a 3D digital SiPM using industrial semiconductor technologies. Proc IEEE Nucl Sci Symp Med Imaging Conf 2018;1:1–4.

75. Gundacker S, Heering A. The silicon photomultiplier: fundamentals and applications of a modern solid-state photon detector. Phys Med Biol 2020;65(17):17TR01.

76. Gola A, Acerbi F, Capasso M, et al. NUV-sensitive silicon photomultiplier technologies developed at Fondazione Bruno Kessler. Sensors 2019;19(2):308.

77. Acerbi F, Gundacker S. Understanding and simulating SiPMs. Nucl Instrum Methods Phys Res 2019;926:16–35.

78. Pratte J-F, Nolet F, Parent S, et al. 3D photon-to-digital converter for radiation instrumentation: motivation and future works. Sensors 2021;21(2):598.

79. Ito M, Hong SJ, Lee JS. Positron emission tomography (PET) detectors with depth-of-interaction (DOI) capability. Biomed Eng Lett 2011;1:70–81.

80. Moses WW, Derenzo SE. Design studies for a PET detector module using a PIN photodiode to measure depth of interaction. IEEE Trans Nucl Sci 1994;41(4):1441–5.

81. Yang Y, Dokhale PA, Silverman RW, et al. Depth of interaction resolution measurements for a high resolution PET detector using position sensitive avalanche photodiodes. Phys Med Biol 2006;51(9):2131.

82. Kang HG, Ko GB, Rhee JT, et al. A dual-ended readout detector using a meantime method for SiPM TOF-DOI PET. IEEE Trans Nucl Sci 2015;62(5):1935–43.

83. Hunter WC, Dewitt DQ, Miyaoka RS. Performance characteristics of a dual-sided position-sensitive sparse-sensor detector for gamma-ray imaging. IEEE Trans Radiat Plasma Med Sci 2021;6(4):385–92.

84. Seo M, Park H, Lee S, et al. Depth-of-interaction positron emission tomography detector with 45° tilted silicon photomultipliers using dual-ended signal readout. Med Phys 2023;50.

85. Zhang Y, Wong W-H. Design study of a practical-entire-torso PET (PET-PET) with low-cost detector designs. Proc IEEE Nucl Sci Symp Med Imaging Conf 2016;1:1–5.

86. Hong SJ, Kwon SI, Ito M, et al. Concept verification of three-layer DOI detectors for small animal PET. IEEE Trans Nucl Sci 2008;55(3):912–7.

87. Liu H, Omura T, Watanabe M, et al. Development of a depth of interaction detector for γ-rays. Nucl Instrum Methods Phys Res 2001;459(1–2):182–90.

88. Zhang N, Thompson CJ, Togane D, et al. Anode position and last dynode timing circuits for dual-layer BGO scintillator with PS-PMT based modular PET detectors. IEEE Trans Nucl Sci 2002;49(5):2203–7.

89. Ito M, Lee JS, Kwon SI, et al. A four-layer DOI detector with a relative offset for use in an animal PET system. IEEE Trans Nucl Sci 2010;57(3):976–81.

90. Goertzen AL, Stortz G, Thiessen JD, et al. First results from a high-resolution small animal SiPM PET insert for PET/MR imaging at 7T. IEEE Trans Nucl Sci 2016;63(5):2424–33.

91. Won JY, Park H, Lee S, et al. Development and initial results of a brain PET insert for simultaneous

7-tesla PET/MRI using an FPGA-only signal digitization method. IEEE Trans Med Imaging 2021; 40(6):1579–90.

92. Kang HG, Tashima H, Wakizaka H, et al. Submillimeter resolution positron emission tomography for high-sensitivity mouse brain imaging. J Nucl Med 2023;64.

93. Tsuda T, Murayama H, Kitamura K, et al. A four-layer depth of interaction detector block for small animal PET. IEEE Trans Nucl Sci 2004;51(5):2537–42.

94. Son JW, Lee MS, Lee JS. A depth-of-interaction PET detector using a stair-shaped reflector arrangement and a single-ended scintillation light readout. Phys Med Biol 2017;62(2):465–83.

95. Yoshida E, Obata F, Kamada K, et al. Development of crosshair light sharing PET detector with TOF and DOI capabilities using fast LGSO scintillator. Phys Med Biol 2021;66(22):225003.

96. Yamamoto S, Ishibashi H. A GSO depth of interaction detector for PET. IEEE Trans Nucl Sci 1998; 45(3):1078–82.

97. Streun M, Brandenburg G, Larue H, et al. Pulse shape discrimination of LSO and LuYAP scintillators for depth of interaction detection in PET. IEEE Trans Nucl Sci 2003;50(3):344–7.

98. Seidel J, Vaquero JJ, Green MV. Resolution uniformity and sensitivity of the NIH ATLAS small animal PET scanner: comparison to simulated LSO scanners without depth-of-interaction capability. IEEE Trans Nucl Sci 2003;50(5):1347–50.

99. Du H, Yang Y, Glodo J, et al. Continuous depth-of-interaction encoding using phosphor-coated scintillators. Phys Med Biol 2009;54(6):1757.

100. Schmall JP, Surti S, Karp JS. Characterization of stacked-crystal PET detector designs for measurement of both TOF and DOI. Phys Med Biol 2015; 60(9):3549–65.

101. Wiener RI, Surti S, Karp JS. DOI determination by rise time discrimination in single-ended readout for TOF PET imaging. IEEE Trans Nucl Sci 2013; 60(3):1478–86.

102. Ko GB, Lee JS. Time-based signal sampling using sawtooth-shaped threshold. Phys Med Biol 2019; 64(12):125020.

103. Chang CM, Cates JW, Levin CS. Time-over-threshold for pulse shape discrimination in a time-of-flight phoswich PET detector. Phys Med Biol 2017;62(1):258–71.

104. Maas MC, Schaart DR, van der Laan DJ, et al. Monolithic scintillator PET detectors with intrinsic depth-of-interaction correction. Phys Med Biol 2009;54(7):1893.

105. Gonzalez-Montoro A, Gonzalez AJ, Pourashraf S, et al. Evolution of PET detectors and event positioning algorithms using monolithic scintillation crystals. IEEE Trans Radiat Plasma Med Sci 2021; 5(3):282–305.

106. Chung YH, Lee S-J, Baek C-H, et al. New design of a quasi-monolithic detector module with DOI capability for small animal pet. Nucl Instrum Methods Phys Res 2008;593(3):588–91.

107. Zhang X, Wang X, Ren N, et al. Performance of long rectangular semi-monolithic scintillator PET detectors. Med Phys 2019;46(4):1608–19.

108. Cucarella N, Barrio J, Lamprou E, et al. Timing evaluation of a PET detector block based on semi-monolithic LYSO crystals. Med Phys 2021;48(12):8010–23.

109. Lewellen TK, Janes M, Miyaoka RS. DMice-a depth-of-interaction detector design for PET scanners. Proc IEEE Nucl Sci Symp Med Imaging Conf 2004;1:2388–92.

110. Ito M, Lee JS, Park M-J, et al. Design and simulation of a novel method for determining depth-of-interaction in a PET scintillation crystal array using a single-ended readout by a multi-anode PMT. Phys Med Biol 2010;55(13):3827.

111. Lee MS, Lee JS. Depth-of-interaction measurement in a single-layer crystal array with a single-ended readout using digital silicon photomultiplier. Phys Med Biol 2015;60(16):6495–514.

112. Miyaoka RS, Lewellen TK, Yu H, et al. Design of a depth of interaction (DOI) PET detector module. IEEE Trans Nucl Sci 1998;45(3):1069–73.

113. Pizzichemi M, Stringhini G, Niknejad T, et al. A new method for depth of interaction determination in PET detectors. Phys Med Biol 2016;61(12):4679.

114. LaBella A, Cao X, Petersen E, et al. High-resolution depth-encoding PET detector module with prismatoid light-guide array. J Nucl Med 2020;61(10): 1528–33.

115. Gundacker S, Martinez Turtos R, Kratochwil N, et al. Experimental time resolution limits of modern SiPMs and TOF-PET detectors exploring different scintillators and Cherenkov emission. Phys Med Biol 2020;65(2):025001.

116. Nadig V, Herweg K, Chou MMC, et al. Timing advances of commercial divalent-ion co-doped LYSO:Ce and SiPMs in sub-100 ps time-of-flight positron emission tomography. Phys Med Biol 2023;68(7):075002.

117. Nemallapudi MV, Gundacker S, Lecoq P, et al. Sub-100 ps coincidence time resolution for positron emission tomography with LSO:Ce codoped with Ca. Phys Med Biol 2015;60(12):4635.

118. Derenzo SE, Choong W-S, Moses WW. Monte Carlo calculations of PET coincidence timing: single and double-ended readout. Phys Med Biol 2015; 60(18):7309.

119. Kwon SI, Roncali E, Gola A, et al. Dual-ended readout of bismuth germanate to improve timing resolution in time-of-flight PET. Phys Med Biol 2019;64(10):105007.

120. Cates JW, Levin CS. Evaluation of a clinical TOF-PET detector design that achieves ≩100 ps

coincidence time resolution. Phys Med Biol 2018; 63(11):115011.

121. Lee MS, Cates JW, Gonzalez-Montoro A, et al. High-resolution time-of-flight PET detector with 100 ps coincidence time resolution using a side-coupled phoswich configuration. Phys Med Biol 2021;66(12):125007.

122. Pourashraf S, Gonzalez-Montoro A, Won JY, et al. Scalable electronic readout design for a 100 ps coincidence time resolution TOF-PET system. Phys Med Biol 2021;66(8):085005.

123. Knapitsch A, Lecoq P. Review on photonic crystal coatings for scintillators. Int J Mod Phys A 2014, 29(30):1430070.

124. Turtos RM, Gundacker S, Polovitsyn A, et al. Ultrafast emission from colloidal nanocrystals under pulsed X-ray excitation. J Inst Met 2016;11(10): P10015.

125. Tomanová K, Čuba V, Brik MG, et al. On the structure, synthesis, and characterization of ultrafast blue-emitting CsPbBr3 nanoplatelets. Apl Mater 2019;7(1):011104.

126. Brunner SE, Schaart DR. BGO as a hybrid scintillator/Cherenkov radiator for cost-effective time-of-flight PET. Phys Med Biol 2017;62(11):4421–39.

127. Kwon SI, Gola A, Ferri A, et al. Bismuth germanate coupled to near ultraviolet silicon photomultipliers for time-of-flight PET. Phys Med Biol 2016;61(18): L38–47.

128. Tao L, He Y, Kanatzidis MG, et al. Study of annihilation photon pair coincidence time resolution using prompt photon emissions in new perovskite bulk crystals. IEEE Trans Radiat Plasma Med Sci 2022;6(7):804–10.

129. Terragni G, Pizzichemi M, Roncali E, et al. Time resolution studies of thallium based Cherenkov semiconductors. Front Phys 2022;10:785627.

130. Cates JW, Levin CS. Electronics method to advance the coincidence time resolution with bismuth germanate. Phys Med Biol 2019;64(17):175016.

131. Catoo JW, Choong WC. Low power implementation of high frequency SiPM readout for Cherenkov and scintillation detectors in TOF-PET. Phys Med Biol 2022;67(19):195009.

132. Efthimiou N, Kratochwil N, Gundacker S, et al. TOF-PET image reconstruction with multiple timing kernels applied on Cherenkov radiation in BGO. IEEE Trans Radiat Plasma Med Sci 2020;5(5): 703–11.

133. Kratochwil N, Gundacker S, Lecoq P, et al. Pushing Cherenkov PET with BGO via coincidence time resolution classification and correction. Phys Med Biol 2020;65(11):115004.

134. Konstantinou G, Lecoq P, Benlloch JM, et al. Metascintillators for ultrafast gamma detectors: a review of current state and future perspectives. IEEE Trans Radiat Plasma Med Sci 2022;6(1):5–15.

135. Turtos RM, Gundacker S, Auffray E, et al. Towards a metamaterial approach for fast timing in PET: experimental proof-of-concept. Phys Med Biol 2019;64(18):185018.

136. Lecoq P. Pushing the limits in time-of-flight PET imaging. IEEE Trans Radiat Plasma Med Sci 2017; 1(6):473–85.

137. Pagano F, Kratochwil N, Salomoni M, et al. Advances in heterostructured scintillators: toward a new generation of detectors for TOF-PET. Phys Med Biol 2022;67(13):135010.

138. Konstantinou G, Latella R, Moliner L, et al. A proof-of-concept of cross-luminescent metascintillators: testing results on a BGO:BaF2 metapixel. Phys Med Biol 2023;68(2):025018.

139. Kang SK, An HJ, Jin H, et al. Synthetic CT generation from weakly paired MR images using cycle-consistent GAN for MR-guided radiotherapy. Biomed Eng Lett 2021;11(3):263–71.

140. Rajendran P, Sharma A, Pramanik M. Photoacoustic imaging aided with deep learning: a review. Biomed Eng Lett 2022;12(2):155–73.

141. Lee MS, Hwang D, Kim JH, et al. Deep-dose: a voxel dose estimation method using deep convolutional neural network for personalized internal dosimetry. Sci Rep 2019;9(1):10308.

142. Rao DKP, Singh R,JV. Automated segmentation of the larynx on computed tomography images: a review. Biomed Eng Lett 2022;12(2):175–83.

143. Liu F, Jang H, Kijowski R, et al. Deep learning MR imaging–based attenuation correction for PET/MR imaging. Radiology 2018;286(2):676–84.

144. Reader AJ, Corda G, Mehranian A, et al. Deep learning for PET image reconstruction. IEEE Trans Radiat Plasma Med Sci 2020;5(1):1–25.

145. Lee JS. A review of deep-learning-based approaches for attenuation correction in positron emission tomography. IEEE Trans Radiat Plasma Med Sci 2021;5(2):160–84.

146. Gong K, Berg E, Cherry SR, et al. Machine learning in PET: from photon detection to quantitative image reconstruction. Proc IEEE 2020;108(1):51–68.

147. Ullah MN, Levin CS. Application of artificial intelligence in PET instrumentation. Pet Clin 2022; 17(1):175–82.

148. Müller F, Schug D, Hallen P, et al. A novel DOI positioning algorithm for monolithic scintillator crystals in PET based on gradient tree boosting. IEEE Trans Radiat Plasma Med Sci 2019;3(4): 465–74.

149. Peng P, Judenhofer MS, Cherry SR. Compton PET: a layered structure PET detector with high performance. Phys Med Biol 2019;64(10):10LT01.

150. Decuyper M, Stockhoff M, Vandenberghe S, et al. Artificial neural networks for positioning of gamma interactions in monolithic PET detectors. Phys Med Biol 2021;66(7):075001.

151. Berg E, Cherry SR. Using convolutional neural networks to estimate time-of-flight from PET detector waveforms. Phys Med Biol 2018;63(2):02LT1.

152. Onishi Y, Hashimoto F, Ote K, et al. Unbiased TOF estimation using leading-edge discriminator and convolutional neural network trained by single-source-position waveforms. Phys Med Biol 2022;67(4):04NT1.

153. Lee S, Lee JS. Inter-crystal scattering recovery of light-sharing PET detectors using convolutional neural networks. Phys Med Biol 2021;66(18):185004.

154. Lee S, Lee JS. Experimental evaluation of convolutional neural network-based inter-crystal scattering recovery for high-resolution PET detectors. Phys Med Biol 2023;68(9):095017.

155. Shim H, Bae S, Lee S, et al. Inter-crystal scattering event identification using a novel silicon photomultiplier signal multiplexing method. Phys Med Biol 2023;68(11):115008.

New Horizons in Brain PET Instrumentation

Magdelena S. Allen, BA[a,b], Michele Scipioni, PhD[a,c], Ciprian Catana, MD, PhD[a,c,*]

KEYWORDS

- Positron emission tomography • Brain PET • Neuroimaging • High spatial resolution
- High sensitivity • Multimodal imaging

KEY POINTS

- Many dedicated brain PET, PET/computed tomography, and PET/magnetic resonance systems are now on or near the commercial market.
- Several standalone PET systems are low cost and have small installation footprints, which combined with adjustable patient positioning configurations increase patient comfort and allow neuroimaging in a variety of new clinical settings.
- With key design features such as scanner geometry, detector design, depth of interaction, time of flight, dedicated brain PET can achieve the highest sensitivity and highest spatial resolution available.
- Dedicated brain PET can enable imaging of small brain structures, low dose imaging, and studies of neurochemical dynamics on short timescales.

INTRODUCTION

PET technology development is often driven by the application of whole-body oncology, but in recent years PET has shown its value as a tool for neuroscience research and clinical applications, including imaging brain metabolism, hemodynamics, protein deposition, neurotransmitter function, receptor binding with high molecular specificity, etc. Dedicated brain PET devices are optimized for neuroimaging, offering higher sensitivity and better spatial resolution than traditional whole-body scanners. This article reviews the design and performance of the state of the art in dedicated brain PET instrumentation.

There exist fundamental physics limits to spatial resolution in PET imaging, such as uncertainties associated with positron range and photon non-collinearity.[1] Dedicated brain scanners can reduce these effects with design features such as magnetic field compatibility to reduce the former and small scanner diameters to reduce the latter. Systems designed for high spatial resolution also employ detectors with novel scintillator crystal configurations. Dedicated brain PET will drive spatial resolution toward to fundamental limits and reduce partial volume effects, enabling more accurate imaging of small brain structures.

Higher spatial resolution necessitates better sensitivity to capture adequate counts per voxel. High sensitivity also opens new frontiers such as low-dose imaging and the imaging of neurochemical dynamics on short timescales. Sensitivity can be improved with dedicated brain scanners via increased solid angle coverage and photon detection efficiency, such as employing novel scanner geometries and detectors with thick scintillator layers to boost attenuation. Of course, thick crystal layers introduce parallax error moving away from the center of the field of view (cFOV), which can be addressed by various methods to encode information about the depth of interaction (DOI) of the photon within the material. Time of flight (TOF) information can further boost the image signal-to-noise ratio (SNR) and contribute to the

[a] Department of Radiology, A. A. Martinos Center for Biomedical Imaging, Massachusetts General Hospital;
[b] Department of Physics, Massachusetts Institute of Technology; [c] Harvard Medical School
* Corresponding author. Department of Radiology, A. A. Martinos Center for Biomedical Imaging, Massachusetts General Hospital.
E-mail address: ccatana@mgh.harvard.edu

PET Clin 19 (2024) 25–36
https://doi.org/10.1016/j.cpet.2023.08.001
1556-8598/24/© 2023 Elsevier Inc. All rights reserved.

effective sensitivity, which is an explanation for why silicon photomultipliers (SiPMs) have become the photon detector of choice even for standalone PET devices.[2] Dedicated brain PET devices also introduce the potential to increase patient comfort, support multifunctional imaging, reduce cost, and reduce installation footprint, increasing accessibility to advanced neuroimaging and opening doors to imaging patients in a variety of new clinical settings. Dedicated brain PET scanners can achieve higher sensitivity and spatial resolution with fewer detector modules and are light weight enough to support adjustable patient positioning (eg, seated or supine) or easy integration as inserts to existing MR imaging systems for simultaneous data acquisition.

Many dedicated brain PET scanners developed with features for high sensitivity, high spatial resolution, increased patient comfort, and reduced siting requirements are now on or near the commercial market. The upcoming sections will discuss these devices, which include those that have been developed as standalone PET and computed tomography (CT) systems, or to serve as MR-compatible inserts for integrated PET/MR imaging. For each category, only the recently developed scanners or those still in development will be discussed, as prior efforts have been described in other review papers (eg, Refs [2,3]). In all categories, the design and performance characteristics of the devices will be summarized, with a particular focus on spatial resolution (reported as full width at half maximum, FWHM), TOF (FWHM), energy resolution (FWHM), sensitivity, and unique features.

STANDALONE PET SYSTEMS

Many standalone dedicated brain PET systems have been developed, offering high sensitivity and high spatial resolution while requiring fewer components to manufacture and thus substantially lowering the cost. They can also have significantly smaller installation footprints than traditional scanners and can support imaging patients in a seated position (4D-PET, CareMiBrain, NeuroLF, and VRAIN; **Fig. 1**) or a variety of adjustable positions (BBX, Pharos, and HIAS-29000; **Fig. 2**). Standalone scanners are also under development to push the limits of spatial resolution (Prism-PET, UHR/scanner approaching in vivo autoradiographic neuro tomography [SAVANT]; **Fig. 3**).

Devices that Allow for Patient Imaging in a Seated Position

The *4D-PET* system was designed by researchers from Polytechnic University of Valencia and Oncovision S.A. (Valencia, Spain) to allow the patient to be imaged in a seated position with eyes uncovered (see **Fig. 1**A). Additional design goals of good spatial resolution, sensitivity, and TOF capabilities are accomplished with semi-monolithic detectors.[4] The 4D-PET system is made up of 320 detector elements, each consisting of an array of 1 × 16 slab-shaped lutetium-yttrium oxyorthosilicate (LYSO) elements (1.6 × 24.2 × 20.0 mm^3) coupled to an array of 8 × 8 silicon photomultipliers (SiPMs). Wedge-like crystals are also placed on both sides of the array. A multiplexing readout electronics system that reduces the number of output signals in a 4:1 ratio makes the system less complex and more cost-effective. The 4D-PET system covers an axial length of 200 mm and has an internal diameter of 280 mm. The configuration of the crystal slabs is crucial for achieving high spatial resolution in the transaxial plane, which is estimated to be around 1 mm in the reconstructed image. This comes at the expense of the axial resolution, which is 2.7 mm. The semi-monolithic crystal allows a DOI resolution of 3.4 mm, with a measured coincidence time resolution (CTR) of 359 ps. The energy resolution is about 10.2% and simulation studies estimate a sensitivity of 16.2% at the cFOV.

The *CareMiBrain* scanner was developed by OncoVision S.A. (Valencia, Spain) for early detection of Alzheimer's disease and other neurologic disorders (see **Fig. 1**B). The CareMiBrain also provides increased patient comfort by imaging the patient in a seated position with eyes uncovered, and boasts a small installation footprint (1.2 × 2.5 m^2) with total cost reduction of 2 to 3 times compared with traditional PET/CT scanners.[5,6] The scanner comprises 3 rings in a cylindrical geometry with 16 detector modules each, with transaxial and axial FOVs of 240 mm and 152 mm, respectively.[7] Each detector module is a 50 × 50 × 15 mm^3 monolith of LYSO coupled to a 12 × 12 array of 2 × 2 mm^2 SiPM pixels (C-Series type from SensL, Ireland), read out by proprietary electronics.[5,8] The DOI resolution afforded by the monolithic detectors and custom readout is 1 mm and the energy resolution is 17%. Average spatial resolution across the radial, tangential, and axial directions is 1.6 mm/1.7 mm at 10 mm/100 mm offset from the cFOV, respectively (NU 2-2012). The sensitivity is 10% at the cFOV (NU 4-2008).[5] Fast and quantitative image reconstruction was achieved with the NiftyPET custom Python package.[7] The device has been technically validated and calibration, acquisition, processing, and reconstruction were optimized with a pilot study with 40 patients, showing comparable performance to standard PET/CT scanners. The device is currently

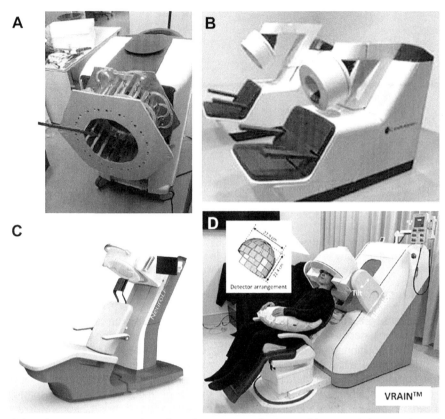

Fig. 1. Standalone brain PET scanners that allow the patient to be imaged in an upright seated position: (*A*) 4D-PET,[4] (*B*) CareMiBrain. (*With permission from* Oncovision.) (*C*) NeuroLF. (*With permission from* Positrigo AG.) and (*D*) VRAIN.[10].

undergoing the second phase of the study to evaluate its clinical utility.[6]

NeuroLF, developed by Positrigo AG (Zurich, Switzerland), is an ultracompact dedicated brain PET system designed to provide comparable image quality to whole-body systems and make functional brain imaging more affordable and comfortable for patients (see **Fig. 1**C). Patients

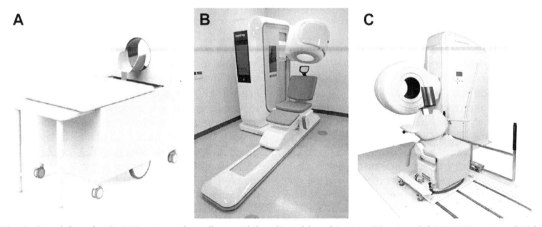

Fig. 2. Standalone brain PET systems that allow widely adjustable subject positioning: (*A*) BBX PET system. (*With permission from* Prescient Medical Imaging.), (*B*) Pharos by Brightonix (image courtesy of Prof. Jae Sung Lee, CEO, Brightonix Imaging Inc.), and (*C*) HIAS-29000. (*With permission from* Hamamatsu Photonics K.K.). These 3 devices are equipped with a patient table designed to switch between chair and bed, allowing imaging of brain, breast, and other peripheral organs.

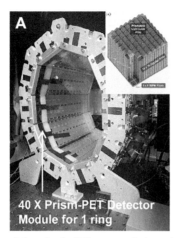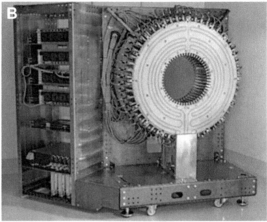

40 X Prism-PET Detector Module for 1 ring

Fig. 3. Standalone brain PET systems designed to achieve best spatial resolution. (*A*) The first single-ring prototype of Prism-PET, developed at Stony Brook University.[15] (*B*) The UHR/SAVANT PET scanner, from a collaboration between University of Sherbrooke and MGH. This research was originally published in JNM. Lecomte R, Normandin M, Tibaudeau C, et al. Scanner Approaching in Vivo Autoradiographic Neuro Tomography (SAVANT): Progress Towards μL Resolution for Imaging the Human Brain. J Nucl Med. 2022;63(supplement 2):2436 LP - 2436. © SNMMI.

are imaged in a seated position and the position of the detector can be adjusted around the head. The PET detectors are positioned in an octagonal prism geometry and the axial FOV is 16.4 cm. Although the complete technical details of the NeuroLF are not yet available, it will be based on the original BPET prototype designed and developed at ETH Zurich (Switzerland).[9] The BPET detector head was composed of detector blocks with 6 × 6 arrays of LYSO crystals bonded to 3 × 3 arrays of SiPMs (Hamamatsu S13360-3050VE). The reported spatial resolution and sensitivity of the BPET were 4.0 mm and 2.9 kcps/kBq, respectively, at the cFOV, and there was no TOF capability. The BPET prototype was successfully used to demonstrate the feasibility of the NeuroLF system for human brain in vivo imaging; however, NeuroLF is expected to provide better spatial and timing resolution.

The first complete brain PET scanner with a hemispherical detector arrangement was developed by investigators from the National Institutes for Quantum Science and Technology (Chiba, Japan) with the goals of providing increased sensitivity scans at lower cost, and is now commercialized in Japan as *VRAIN* (see **Fig. 1**D). The current prototype has 54 detectors, with 45 in a hemispherical arrangement and 9 more to supplement coverage along the back of the neck. The inner diameter of the bottom detector ring is 279 mm and the maximum axial FOV is 224 mm. Each detector is a 12 × 12 array of chemically polished 4.1 × 4.1 × 10 mm³ lutetium fine silicate crystals coupled 1:1 to a 12 × 12 array of SiPMs (S13361 series, Hamamatsu Photonics, K.K.) of 4 × 4 mm² active area. Detectors are read out with a customized C13500 series module from

Hamamatsu Photonics K. K.[10] Performance tests show spatial resolution of 2.8 mm/3.6 mm at 1 cm/10 cm offset from the cFOV, resulting in clear separation of 2.2 mm rods.[10] The TOF resolution is 256 ps, a dramatic improvement compared with the 20 ns reported for the first prototype.[11] The measured sensitivity is 4.2 kcps/MBq and increases to 25 kcps/MBq after TOF gain. FDG imaging has been demonstrated in healthy human volunteers showing the whole brain with high contrast and without artifact, and resolving small deep brain nuclei (eg, the inferior colliculus, red nucleus, and substantia nigra).[12]

Devices that Allow Widely Adjustable Subject Positioning

Brain, Breast, eXtremities (BBX) PET system was developed by Prescient Imaging (Hawthorne, CA, USA) as a portable scanner that can be adjusted to allow for brain imaging in a seated position, breast imaging in a prone position, and extremity imaging in other positions (see **Fig. 2**A). The BBX PET scanner was also designed to fit through standard doors and elevators and weighs only about 225 kg. The detectors consist of double-layer staggered lutetium fine silicate (LFS) crystals, with 13 × 13 and 14 × 14 arrays and a 1.76 mm pitch, coupled to multi-pixel photon counters (MPPCs) and readout electronics. The scanner is a ring of 128 blocks with 25 cm and 10 cm transaxial and axial imaging FOVs, respectively. Preliminary evaluation shows spatial resolution of approximately 2.2 mm and a total efficiency of 1.1%.

Pharos is a multipurpose brain PET scanner developed by Brightonix in South Korea (see

Fig. 2B). The scanner can be rotated 180°, and the patient table is designed to switch between chair and bed, allowing 4+ different scanning modes for brain, breast, and other peripheral organs. The detector comprises 4 rings of diameter 33 cm and has a maximum axial FOV of 26.2 cm. Each ring consists of 20 sectors each containing 3 × 12 block detectors. Every detector is an 8 × 8 lutetium-based scintillator array with 2.0 mm crystal pitch is 2.0 mm and 15 mm thickness, with two 4 × 4 SiPM arrays coupled to both sides of the crystal array. This dual-sided readout provides DOI encoding from the ratio of the pulse integrals.

The *HIAS-29000* is a dedicated brain TOF-PET scanner developed by Hamamatsu Photonics K.K. (Hamamatsu, Japan) with a gantry allowing for a variety of patient positions during imaging including seated and supine (see **Fig. 2**C). The HIAS-29000 consists of 28 units in a cylindrical geometry, each housing 4 detector modules, with transaxial and axial FOVs of 360 mm and 230 mm, respectively. Each module is a 16 × 16 LFS crystals of 3.14 × 3.14 × 20 mm^3 coupled 1:1 to a 16 × 16 array of SiPM pixels of 3 × 3 mm^2 active area, with proprietary readout electronics optimized for TOF. The system is also equipped with a motion correction system that monitors patient movement with a camera and reflective markers placed on the patient's head.[13] The TOF resolution was 280 ps. Average spatial resolution was under 4 mm up to 100 mm offset from the cFOV, with average resolution of 2.2 mm at 10 mm offset position. With the motion correction system, an average spatial resolution of 5.1 mm at 100 mm offset in the FOV could be achieved even with ±15 mm of translation and ±7° of rotation. In the motion correction system performance evaluation, the average spatial resolution was 2.7 mm at 10 mm offset position with a point source translating ±15 mm along the y-axis during acquisition, and successfully recovered similar quality to an at-rest image of a Hoffman phantom as well.[13]

Devices Designed to Achieve Best Spatial Resolution

The *Prism-PET* scanner developed at Stony Brook University (Stony Brook, NY, USA) images subjects in a supine position with the primary goal of high spatial resolution (see **Fig. 3**A). The scanner geometry conforms to the ellipse of the human head in the axial plane, allowing fewer detector modules to be used while achieving high solid angle coverage and high sensitivity, and characterization of a prototype with a single ring of 40 modules has been completed. The ring has an axial FOV of 25.5 mm, short diameter of 29.1 cm,

and long diameter of 38.5 mm. Each module contains 16 × 16 LYSO crystals (1.5 × 1.5 × 20 mm^3) which are 4:1 coupled to an 8 × 8 SiPM array with pixels of 3 × 3 mm^2. A segmented light guide comprising right triangular prisms opposite the SiPMs confines light sharing to nearest-neighbor crystals and is optimized for crystal identification and DOI encoding. Data are acquired with front-end TOF modules developed by PETsys Electronics.[14] The prototype achieved a DOI resolution of 2.85 mm FWHM, energy resolution of 12.6%, TOF resolution of 271 ps, and peak absolute sensitivity of 1.2%. The average spatial resolution is 1.53 mm across the entire FOV, and tests with Derenzo phantoms show spatial resolution of less than 2 mm. Tests with Hoffman brain phantoms and custom brain slice phantoms including small nuclei show the ability to accurately resolve brain structures 2 to 3 mm in diameter.[15] Future work includes expanding the prototype to 10 rings of modules, facilitated by a multiplexing approach, and inclusion of a newly developed wearable motion tracking and correction system with 6 degrees of freedom.[16,17]

The *ultra-high resolution (UHR) PET brain scanner* was designed at the University of Sherbrooke (Sherbrooke, QC, Canada; see **Fig. 3**B).[18] It is based on the LabPET II technology previously used for building a high spatial resolution preclinical PET scanner and images patients supine with the primary goal of improving the intrinsic spatial resolution.[18] The scanner is composed of 1008 detector modules consisting of 4 detectors each composed of 1.12 × 1.12 × 12 mm^3 LYSO crystals one-to-one coupled to 4 × 8 avalanche photodiode arrays. The axial FOV is 235 mm, and the ring diameter is 390 mm. In collaboration with investigators from the Gordon Center, MGH and funded by the NIH BRAIN Initiative, the Sherbrooke team is developing a version of this scanner with DOI capabilities called SAVANT.[19] The target spatial resolution is 1.25 mm FWHM at the cFOV and 2.1 mm at 10 cm offset from the cFOV. The expected sensitivity is 5%.

PET-COMPUTED TOMOGRAPHY SYSTEM

A next-generation dedicated brain PET/CT imaging system has also been recently developed by Yale, UC Davis, and United Imaging with the goal of achieving ultra-high sensitivity (10 times higher than the siemens high resolution research tomograph, HRRT), high spatial resolution (<2 mm across the human brain), and continuous head motion correction (**Fig. 4**). This effort was partially supported by NIH BRAIN Initiative. Inspired by the whole-body uEXPLORER, the NeuroEXPLORER

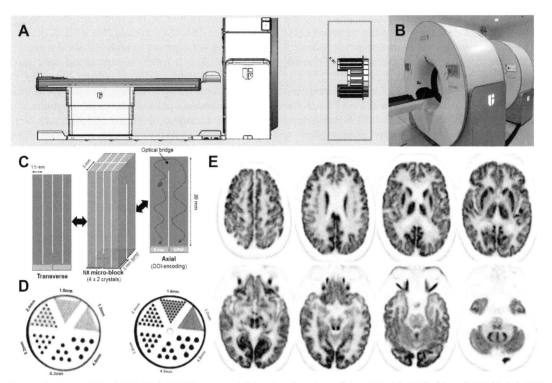

Fig. 4. The NeuroEXPLORER (NX) PET/CT system: (*A*) Design drawing of the NX with CT (left) and PET (right). PET detector array shown on the right with shoulder cutouts to center brain in axial field of view. (*B*) Constructed NX system. (*C*) Detector design showing NX microblock with DOI encoding with an optical bridge and dual SiPM readout. (*D*) Mini-deluxe phantom images reconstructed with TOF and DOI OSEM with 8 iterations (left) and 50 iterations (right); 10 subsets in each. (*E*) First human brain FDG images demonstrating exceptionally high resolution in the cortex and subcortical structures. (Images courtesy of Richard Carson, PhD, Yale School of Medicine PET Center.)

(NX) scanner has an extended axial FOV of 49.5 cm (see **Fig. 4**A, B).[20] A partial detector ring with a shoulder cut-out enhances sensitivity by allowing the brain to be positioned at the cFOV and enables image-derived input function estimation from the carotid arteries. The NX uses a novel U-shaped light-sharing microblock detector consisting of a 4 × 2 array of 1.56 × 3.07 × 20 mm³ LYSO crystals coupled to a 2 × 2 arrays of 3 × 3 mm² SiPMs (see **Fig. 4**C). An optical bridge between adjacent crystals allows the light to be shared between SiPMs in the axial direction, enabling single-ended DOI encoding and intercrystal scatter detection. The NX has a total of 16,416 microblocks arranged in 20 detector modules that form a cylindrical detector ring with a diameter of 52.4 cm. Recent evaluation shows sensitivity of 46.8 kcps/MBq, transverse spatial resolution of 1.8/2.2 mm at 0/10-cm offset from the cFOV, TOF resolution of 236 ps, and energy resolution of 10.5%. The peak noise eqiuvalent counts (NEC) rate was 1.3 kcps at an activity concentration of 57.5 kBq/cc (see **Fig. 4**D). The team

also recently performed the first human scan with the NX scanner and an initial comparison with the Siemens Biograph Vision PET/CT scanner, and the NX demonstrates exquisite spatial resolution clearly superior to the Vision (see **Fig. 4**E). They plan to further develop the system by implementing continuous motion correction and conducting comprehensive comparisons with the Vision and HRRT systems.

MR-COMPATIBLE PET INSERTS

Several dedicated brain PET devices have been designed as inserts to existing MR systems for simultaneous imaging. The PETcoil and Cubresa BrainPET are 3-T MR-compatible inserts (**Fig. 5**), and the Gachon University BrainPET, UHF BrainPET, and HSTR-BrainPET are 7-T MR-compatible inserts (**Fig. 6**).

3-T MR-compatible PET Inserts

Researchers from Stanford focused on designing a cost-efficient TOF PET insert that can be

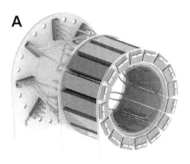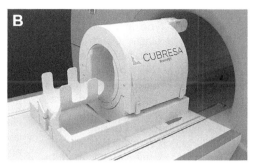

Fig. 5. 3-T MR-compatible PET inserts: (A) PET Coil System. (*With permission from* PETcoil, Inc.) and (B) Cubresa BrainPET (image courtesy of Cubresa Inc.).

integrated with any 3T MR system called the *PETcoil* (see **Fig. 5**A).[21] To reduce interference between the 2 modalities, the radiofrequency (RF)-penetrable PET insert electrically floats relative to the MR imaging system via 1-mm air gaps placed between adjacent shielded PET detector modules. Non-magnetic batteries are used to power the PET camera so it is electrically uncoupled from the MR system. Thus, instead of requiring dedicated RF coils, the standard MR body coil can be used to transmit and receive the RF signal through the gaps between the PET modules, although improved MR performance was subsequently demonstrated when positioning the receive coil

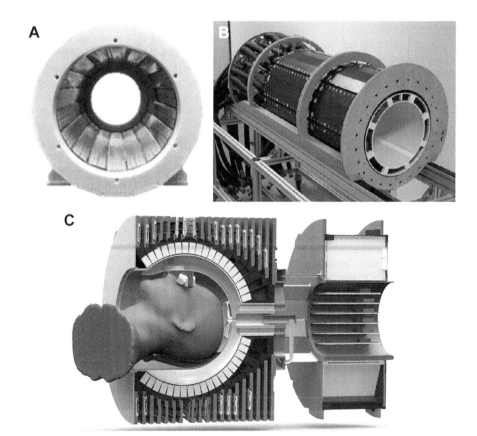

Fig. 6. 7-T MR-compatible PET inserts: (A) The Gachon University BrainPET,[26] (B) the UHF BrainPET, and (C) the HDNCC. The rendering of the HDNCC insert highlights the effort in maximizing solid angle coverage of the brain by adopting a spherical geometry. ([B] Image courtesy of Dr. Christoph Lerche, Forschungszentrum Jülich GmbH, Germany)

inside the insert.[22] The PETcoil detector modules are shielded with a new type of Faraday cage created by 3D printing a plastic enclosure and spraying a conductive layer of silver-coated copper flakes suspended in acrylic lacquer. The PET insert consists of 16 detector modules arranged in a cylindrical geometry and a phased array receive coil, with each detector module having 6 submodules. The submodules consist of 128 SiPMs coupled to LYSO crystals and an application-specific integrated circuit (ASIC) readout board. There are 2-mm gaps between adjacent detector modules on the inner diameter of the PET ring to promote RF-penetrability. The axial FOV of the system is 160 mm. Promising results were recently reported using 2 fully assembled PET detector modules both in terms of PET performance (eg, 242 ps timing resolution and 2.74 mm intrinsic spatial resolution) and lack of interference with the MR system.[23,24]

The *Cubresa BrainPET* is another 3T MR-compatible PET insert that has recently been developed by Cubresa, Inc (Winnipeg, Canada; see **Fig. 5**B). The BrainPET is vendor-agnostic and can be incorporated into any clinical MR system with a minimum bore size of 60 cm. The design is based on Cubresa's established NuPET 66 insert that was first developed for the preclinical market.[25] The new BrainPET has an axial FOV of 200 mm and incorporates an ergonomic head holder which allows the insert to slide into place over the patient for imaging. The PET detector modules consist of dual-layer offset LYSO scintillator arrays (bottom layer 26 × 12 crystals, 2.35 × 2.35 × 12 mm; top layer 25 x 11 crystals, 2.35 × 2.35 × 8 mm) coupled to SiPMs (Array-J 30035, Onsemi Scottsdale, AZ, USA). The expected performance characteristics for the Cubresa BrainPET include sub-2 mm spatial resolution and 8% sensitivity. The BrainPET contains an actively decoupled quadrature-polarized transmit coil and helmet-shaped 32-channel receive array. The system includes an MR-conditional, EMI-quiet PET electronics cabinet that resides within the MR suite and connects via fiber to the BrainPET workstation, which resides in the MR console room and runs Cubresa's proprietary data acquisition and image reconstruction software. The Cubresa BrainPET is noteworthy in its streamlined, removable design offering a lightweight, portable PET insert solution that occupies a small footprint within the MR suite. The BrainPET also includes an MR-compatible device that lifts the insert to the MR imaging bore for installation and use, and easily removes and stores the insert away from the scanner when PET/MR imaging is complete to support multiuse imaging workflows within an MR imaging facility.

7-T MR-compatible PET Inserts

At *Gachon University (South Korea), a* brain PET insert was developed for integration with the Siemens 7T Magnetom MR scanner (see **Fig. 6**A). The PET detector block consists of a 2-layer lutetium oxyorthosilicate (LSO) array coupled to a 2 × 2 array of 4 × 4 SiPMs (S13361-3050NE-04, Hamamatsu Photonics K.K). The upper scintillator layer is a 11 × 11 array of 2.09 × 2.09 × 8 mm^3 and the lower one is a 12 × 12 array of 2.09 × 2.09 × 12 mm^3. Up to 16 detector blocks in a 2 × 8 configuration can be grouped together in sectors and 18 of these sectors make up a PET insert with an inner diameter of 33 cm and transaxial FOV of 25.6 cm. A 2 × 6 detector blocks version of the insert that provides an axial coverage of 16.7 cm was built and evaluated in a first stage. The spatial resolution at the cFOV is 2.5 mm, the sensitivity is 6.19%, and high-quality images were obtained using phantoms both outside and inside the MR scanner.[26]

Within the Helmholtz Validation Fund Project "Next generation BrainPET scanner for 7T MRI", a UHF-MR imaging compatible BrainPET insert prototype for dedicated human neuroimaging is being developed and built (see **Fig. 6**B). The insert was designed to achieve at least 12% sensitivity at isocenter, a homogeneous spatial image resolution of 1.5 to 2.0 mm over the whole brain, a CTR of 500 ps, and an axial FOV of 24 cm. A staggered layer pixelated scintillation detector design was chosen for the 120 scintillation block detectors (5 rings with 24 detector blocks).[27] Three layers 7/8/9 mm thick of LSO scintillator with 24 × 24/23 × 24/ 22 × 23 pixels of 2.0 mm pitch, respectively, are coupled with a light guide to a 12 × 12-channels digital SiPM to form a detector unit. The detectors are read out by MR-compatible electronics shielded with carbon fiber-reinforced plastic, and SiPMs and PET module electronics are thermally stabilized with an MR-compatible liquid cooling system.[28] Light sharing and a machine learning positioning algorithm will be used for crystal identification and energy estimation.[29] Image reconstruction will be done with PET reconstruction software toolkit (PRESTO), a maximum likelihood expectation-maximization (ML-EM)-based image reconstruction toolkit.[30] Monte Carlo simulations with GATE assessed sensitivity and spatial resolution, finding 12% sensitivity at the isocenter when simulating a low activity source and spatial resolution below 2.0 mm over the whole human brain when simulating a Derenzo phantom with 20 cm diameter. A highly PET-transparent, multi-channel transmit/receive coil array has been designed and built for use with the BrainPET insert.[31]

Finally, the authors and their colleagues from the MGH Martinos Center, with collaborators from Siemens, Hamamatsu, University of Tuebingen, Complutense University of Madrid, and University of Texas at Arlington, are currently developing the Human Dynamic Neuro-Chemical Connectome (HDNCC) scanner (see **Fig. 6**C). This project is supported by the NIH BRAIN initiative. This system is a high-spatiotemporal resolution dedicated brain PET insert (*HSTR-BrainPET*) that can be integrated with the commercially available 7T Siemens Magnetom Terra and the original 7T Magnetom prototype, both available at the Martinos Center, for the investigation of neurochemical dynamics.[3,32] The patient is imaged supine and visual and audio stimuli will be provided with a low-profile wearable MR-compatible system. Unlike the other scanners discussed above, the HSTR-BrainPET is not targeted toward commercialization, and thus has relatively more freedom from typical economic constraints to employ additional design features for maximizing sensitivity. Using high-performance detectors in a novel geometry with high solid angle coverage, the project aims to increase the PET sensitivity by an order of magnitude compared with existing PET systems to study neurochemical-specific brain activation on short timescales comparable to those of functional MR imaging. Design goals include high spatial resolution (targeting 1–2 mm), DOI capability, good TOF performance, and excellent sensitivity (25% intrinsic sensitivity, with additional gain expected from TOF), for an order-of-magnitude increase compared with existing systems. The HSTR-BrainPET scanner will achieve unprecedented solid angle coverage with 872 detectors in 19 rings with a maximum inner diameter of 32 cm. The detectors will be progressively angled within the rings to form a spherical geometry around the head, and each detector is a 10 × 10 array of 1.6 × 1.6 × 26 mm LSO crystals manufactured by Siemens coupled to a 4 × 4 SiPM array with 4 × 4 mm² pixels (Hamamatsu Photonics, S13546H series) read out by custom electronics from Hamamatsu. Crystal position will be extracted through Anger logic, allowing the spatial resolution to be set by crystal rather than SiPM pixel size, and DOI information will be obtained from the light-sharing characteristics of the array. A high-performance transmit-receive RF coil is being developed in house to be integrated with the HSTR-BrainPET.

WHAT RECENT TRENDS TELL US ABOUT THE FUTURE

Advancements of PET imaging technology are vital to furthering our understanding of the human brain, from studying neurochemical dynamics to early detection of pathologic changes associated with neurodegenerative diseases. The latest generation dedicated brain scanners provide the means to image the brain with higher sensitivity and spatial resolution than ever before and their commercialization can offer many advantages for patient comfort and clinical adoption.

Standalone dedicated organ scanners can potentially improve access to PET imaging by lowering the cost and siting requirements. In previous years, most dedicated brain PET devices were developed in academia, and few made it to the commercial market, never being broadly adopted for clinical use. Today, most of the scanners discussed above were spearheaded by small companies founded specifically to develop dedicated brain PET technology or in collaboration with industrial partners, and are or will soon be commercially available. A design goal for many of these scanners is to increase patient comfort by enabling imaging in nonsupine positions. The 4D-PET, CareMiBrain, NeuroLF, and VRAIN scanners allow imaging in a seated position, some with eyes uncovered. The BBX, HIAS-29000, and Pharos scanners allow widely adjustable positioning, which also facilitates imaging of other body parts (eg, breast, extremity). These developments have made PET hardware more affordable and user- and patient-friendly, which combined with the increasing availability of clinically useful radiotracers that do not require on-site cyclotron or radiochemistry expertise will make PET imaging available to a larger number of patients and in different clinical scenarios (eg, at patient bedside, in the operating room, etc.).

Several scanners have been specifically designed as upgrades to the HRRT, a scanner that has been used for numerous studies over the last 2 decades.[33] This increased spatial resolution was achieved with scintillator crystal arrays that are finely segmented or employ monolithic or semi-monolithic geometries, and by reducing the noncollinearity effects due to the small diameter of dedicated scanners. To reduce the image degradation across the FOV due to parallax error introduced by crystal thickness in small-diameter scanners, a variety of DOI methods (eg, layered detectors, dual-readout, light sharing between crystals, semi-monolithic detectors, etc.) have been employed.[33] Equally important, the developers of several of the scanners (eg, NX, HIAS-29000, UHR/SAVANT, HSTR-BrainPET) have proposed advanced approaches for head motion correction to minimize subject-related image blurring. All of these advances will enable neuroscientists and clinical researchers to delve into the advantages of higher-spatial-resolution PET imaging, including the unprecedented identification of small brain structures such as nuclei 1 to 2 mm in size.

Improving spatial resolution must be accompanied by similar advances in sensitivity to ensure adequate counts are collected per resolution element. In addition to reducing the scanner diameter and using thick crystals to improve the sensitivity, the solid angle coverage was dramatically increased either by using noncylindrical geometries (VRAIN, HSTR-BrainPET) or extending the axial FOV (NX). TOF can further increase effective sensitivity. Thus, dedicated brain scanners with up to an order of magnitude higher effective sensitivity will soon be available and are expected to open new avenues for PET imaging, including low-dose imaging, fast data acquisition, advanced kinetic modeling, high-temporal-resolution imaging of neurotransmitter function dynamics, and assessment of metabolic processes/protein accumulation at pico- to nanomolar concentrations. To give just a few examples, these breakthroughs could facilitate early disease detection, repeated examinations or scanning younger subjects with minimal radiation exposure, and direct monitoring of drug effects.

Except for the NX scanner, all devices discussed do not rely on CT data acquired during the same examination for attenuation correction. Substantial progress has been made in generating attenuation maps with highly accurate MR-based approaches as well as using deep learning-enabled methods that use exclusively the PET data collected with many of the clinically relevant radiotracers for this purpose.[34–37] Similarly, deep learning approaches can also be used to perform scatter and partial volume corrections. Deep learning-based scatter correction approaches can surpass the accuracy of single scatter simulations while boasting shorter processing times than both single scatter correction and Monte Carlo simulations.[38] Standard partial volume correction methods rely on coregistered and segmented of MR or CT data. Algorithms trained with these data can then perform partial volume corrections on PET data without the need for additional anatomic information and have been shown to perform well across scanners, radiotracers, and pathologies. Deep learning-driven corrections have great potential to improve the quality of the PET images and facilitate the use of standalone PET scanners in a variety of clinical and research settings.[39] Finally, progress has continued to be made in the development of MR-compatible brain PET inserts both for 3-T and high-field MR systems. Although compatibility with high-field MR presents more technical challenges, it also provides higher resolution anatomic or functional hemodynamic data. Simultaneous acquisition provides improved spatiotemporal correlation of PET functional data and MR anatomic data and better diagnostic clinical performance, and it opens doors to study brain metabolism in new ways. Uniquely, the HSTR-BrainPET is optimized for novel studies in basic neuroscience, and is designed for unprecedented sensitivity, high spatial resolution, and 7-T MR compatibility. These features will both advance longitudinal studies (eg, low-dose repeated scans in progressive disease and coregistration with high resolution anatomic MR imaging) and breakground in dynamic assessment of neurochemical-specific brain activation on timescales comparable to functional MR imaging (and with the simultaneous acquisition functional MR imaging data), with countless applications to drug response, addiction, psychiatric disease, and neurodegenerative diseases.

SUMMARY

Significant advancements in dedicated brain PET instrumentation have been made over the past few years, surpassing previous standards for sensitivity and spatial resolution. Many standalone brain PET devices optimized for clinical neuroimaging are close to or already on the commercial market. Some boast unprecedented affordability and flexibility for installation and patient positioning, and others have been optimized for high spatial resolution for imaging small brain structures. PET/CT and integrated PET/MR systems are also under development promising high resolution data and improved co-registration of spatiotemporal data between modalities. Dedicated brain PET technology is yielding the highest sensitivity and highest spatial resolution neuroimaging available, with a focus on lowering barriers to adoption in the clinical setting, and will push continue to push advancements in disease detection and basic neuroscience.

FUNDING

This work was supported, in part, by BRAIN Initiative NIH-NIBIB & NINDS grant 1U01EB029826-01, NSF Graduate Research Fellowship, and Peskoff Physics Fellowship awarded by the Department of Physics, MIT.

DISCLOSURE

The authors have no conflicts of interest to disclose.

REFERENCES

1. Moses WW. Fundamental limits of spatial resolution in PET. Nucl Instruments Methods Phys Res Sect A Accel Spectrometers, Detect Assoc Equip 2011; 648:S236–40.
2. Majewski S. The path to the "ideal" brain PET imager: the race is on, the role for TOF PET. Nuovo Cim della Soc Ital di Fis C 2020;43(1):1–35.
3. Catana C. Development of dedicated brain PET imaging devices: recent advances and future perspectives. J Nucl Med 2019;60(8):1044–52.
4. Gonzaloz Montoro A, Barbera J, Sanchez D, et al. A new brain dedicated PET scanner with 4D detector information. Bio Algorithm Med Syst 2022;18(1):107–19.
5. Moliner L, Rodríguez-Alvarez MJ, Catret JV, et al. NEMA Performance Evaluation of CareMiBrain dedicated brain PET and Comparison with the whole-body and dedicated brain PET systems. Sci Rep 2019;9(1):1–10.
6. Cabrera-Martín MN, González-Pavón G, Sanchís Hernández M, et al. Validation technique and improvements introduced in a new dedicated brain positron emission tomograph (CareMiBrain). Rev Española Med Nucl e Imagen Mol (English Ed. 2021;40(4):239–48.
7. Morera-Ballester C, Jiménez-Serrano S, Beschwitz S, et al. NiftyPET: Fast Quantitative Image Reconstruction for a New Brain PET Camera CareMiBrain. IEEE; 2021. p. 1–3.
8. González-Montoro A, Sánchez F, Martí R, et al. Detector block performance based on a monolithic LYSO crystal using a novel signal multiplexing method. Nucl Instruments Methods Phys Res Sect A Accel Spectrometers, Detect Assoc Equip. 2018;912:372–7.
9. Ahnen ML, Fischer J, Kuegler N, et al. Performance of the ultra-compact fully integrated brain PET system BPET. IEEE; 2020. p. 1–4.
10. Akamatsu G, Takahashi M, Tashima H, et al. Performance evaluation of VRAIN: a brain dedicated PET with a hemispherical detector arrangement. Phys Med Biol 2022;67(22). https://doi.org/10.1088/1361-6560/ac9e87.
11. Tashima H, Yoshida E, Iwao Y, et al. First prototyping of a dedicated PET system with the hemisphere detector arrangement. Phys Med Biol 2019;64(6). https://doi.org/10.1088/1361-6560/ab012c.
12. Takahashi M, Akamatsu G, Iwao Y, et al. Small nuclei identification with a hemispherical brain PET. EJNMMI Phys 2022;9(1). https://doi.org/10.1186/s40658-022-00498-4.
13. Onishi Y, Isobe T, Ito M, et al. Performance evaluation of dedicated brain PET scanner with motion correction system. Ann Nucl Med 2022;36(8):746–55.
14. Francesco A Di, Bugalho R, Oliveira L, et al. TOF-PET2: a high-performance ASIC for time and amplitude measurements of SiPM signals in time-of-flight applications. J Instrum 2016;11(03):C03042.
15. Zeng X, Wang Z, Tan W, et al. A conformal TOF–DOI Prism-PET prototype scanner for high-resolution quantitative neuroimaging. Med Phys 2023. https://doi.org/10.1002/mp.16223.
16. LaBella A, Petersen E, Cao X, et al. 36-to-1 multiplexing with prism-PET for high resolution TOF-DOI PET. J Nucl Med 2021;62(supplement 1). 38 LP. Available at: http://jnm.snmjournals.org/content/62/supplement_1/38.abstract.
17. Tan W, Wang Z, Zeng X, et al. Wearable electromagnetic motion tracking with submillimeter accuracy: an experimental study using high-resolution Prism-PET brain scanner. J Nucl Med 2022;63(supplement 2). 3320 LP. Available at: http://jnm.snmjournals.org/content/63/supplement_2/3320.abstract.
18. Gaudin E, Toussaint M, Thibaudeau C, et al. Performance simulation of an Ultrahigh resolution brain PET scanner using 1.2-mm pixel detectors. IEEE Trans Radiat Plasma Med Sci 2019;3(3):334–42.
19. Lecomte R, Normandin M, Tibaudeau C, et al. Scanner approaching in vivo Autoradiographic Neuro tomography (SAVANT): progress towards μL resolution for imaging the human brain. J Nucl Med 2022;63(supplement 2). 2436 LP. Available at: http://jnm.snmjournals.org/content/63/supplement_2/2436.abstract.
20. Cherry SR, Jones T, Karp JS, et al. Total-body PET: maximizing sensitivity to create new opportunities for clinical research and patient care. J Nucl Med 2018;59(1):3–12.
21. Grant AM, Lee BJ, Chang C-M, et al. Simultaneous PET/MR imaging with a radio frequency-penetrable PET insert. Med Phys 2017;44(1):112–20.
22. Lee BJ, Watkins RD, Lee KS, et al. Performance evaluation of RF coils integrated with an RF-penetrable PET insert for simultaneous PET/MRI. Magn Reson Med 2019;81(2):1434–46.
23. Dong Q, Chang C-M, Lee BJ, et al. The PETcoil project: PET performance evaluation of two detector modules for a second generation RF-penetrable TOF-PET brain dedicated insert for simultaneous PET/MRI. Phys Med Biol 2023;68(8):85010.
24. Dong Q, Adams Z, Watkins RD, et al. Study of compatibility between a 3T MR system and detector modules for a second generation RF-penetrable TOF-PET insert for simultaneous PET/MRI. Med Phys 2023. https://doi.org/10.1002/mp.16354.
25. Cubresa NuPET. Available at: https://www.cubresa.com/products/nupet/. Accessed April 5, 2023.
26. Won JY, Park H, Lee S, et al. Development and initial results of a brain PET insert for simultaneous 7-Tesla PET/MRI using an FPGA-only signal Digitization method. IEEE Trans Med Imaging 2021;40(6):1579–90.

27. Ito M., Hong S.J., Lee J.S., et al., Four-layer DOI detector with a relative offset in animal PET system. In 2007 IEEE Nuclear Science Symposium Conference Record, Vol. 6, 2007, IEEE. 4296-4299.

28. Weissler D, Dey T, Gebhardt P, et al. Hyperion III – a flexible PET detector platform for simultaneous PET/MRI. Nuklearmedizin 2020;59(02):V93.

29. Lerche CW, Salomon A, Goldschmidt B, et al. Maximum likelihood positioning and energy correction for scintillation detectors. Phys Med Biol 2016; 61(4):1650.

30. Scheins JJ, Vahedipour K, Pietrzyk U, et al. High performance volume-of-intersection projectors for 3D-PET image reconstruction based on polar symmetries and SIMD vectorisation. Phys Med Biol 2015;60(24):9349.

31. Choi C-H, Hong S-M, Felder J, et al. A novel J-Shape Antenna array for simultaneous MR-PET or MR-SPECT imaging. IEEE Trans Med Imaging 2022; 41(5):1104–13.

32. Scipioni M., Corbeil J., Allen M.S., et al., Design and Development of the Human Dynamic NeuroChemical Connectome Scanner. In: IEEE Nucler Science Symposium and Medical Imaging Conference, November 4-11, Vancouver, Canada; 2023.

33. Wienhard K, Schmand M, Casey ME, et al. The ECAT HRRT: performance and first clinical application of the new high resolution research tomograph. IEEE Trans Nucl Sci 2002;49(1 I):104–10.

34. Catana C. Attenuation correction for human PET/MRI studies. Phys Med Biol 2020;65(23):23TR02.

35. Minoshima S, Cross D. Application of artificial intelligence in brain molecular imaging. Ann Nucl Med 2022;36(2):103–10.

36. Hashimoto F, Ito M, Ote K, et al. Deep learning-based attenuation correction for brain PET with various radiotracers. Ann Nucl Med 2021;35(6): 691–701.

37. Arabi H, Bortolin K, Ginovart N, et al. Deep learning-guided joint attenuation and scatter correction in multitracer neuroimaging studies. Hum Brain Mapp 2020;41(13):3667–79.

38. Laurent B, Bousse A, Merlin T, et al. PET scatter estimation using deep learning U-Net architecture. Phys Med Biol 2023;68(6). https://doi.org/10.1088/1361-6560/ac9a97.

39. Sanaat A, Shooli H, Böhringer AS, et al. A cycle-consistent adversarial network for brain PET partial volume correction without prior anatomical information. Eur J Nucl Med Mol Imaging 2023;50(7): 1881–96.

Advances in Breast PET Instrumentation

Srilalan Krishnamoorthy, PhD*, Suleman Surti, PhD

KEYWORDS

- Breast cancer • Positron emission tomography • PET • PEM • Breast PET • Dedicated breast PET
- High spatial resolution • Small lesion

KEY POINTS

- Dedicated Breast PET scanners provide higher spatial resolution and sensitivity compared with whole-body PET scanners.
- Temporal resolution improvement of PET detectors has the potential to improve PET image quality and permit the design of scanner geometries which permit quantitative imaging without compromising its integration within the clinic.
- Development of novel breast cancer-specific PET radiotracers which help in biological characterization of breast tumor lesions have unlocked several exciting applications including guiding and monitoring treatment and therapy response.
- Commercial availability of dedicated breast PET scanners over the past decade will help in evaluating its potential for a wider role in breast cancer.

ROLE OF PET IMAGING IN BREAST CANCER

Breast cancer (BC) is the most prevalent form of cancer in women and recently has surpassed lung cancer as the most diagnosed cancer.[1] According to references[1,2], approximately 12% of women globally are likely to develop some form of BC in the course of their lifetime. Early diagnosis increases the probability of treatment success.[3] Medical imaging is noninvasive and plays a critical role in screening, detection, treatment, and management of BC. Mammography has very high sensitivity for detecting lesions and is the most commonly used imaging modality for BC screening. Despite several technical advances and the advent of digital breast tomosynthesis (DBT),[4,5] it however has lower specificity that is, the ability to differentiate between malignant and benign tumors.[6,7] Mammographic sensitivity is also lower for women with dense breasts, and ultrasound imaging has been approved as an adjunct imaging modality for such cases. Mammography, ultrasound, and breast-MRI thus constitute the bulk of screening and diagnostic scans for breast imaging.[8,9]

PET, using appropriate biomarkers, has the capability to provide information about tumor biology. This information can provide very high specificity in differentiating malignancy. However, the tumor biology information from PET is complementary to anatomic information obtained from other imaging modalities like mammography, computed tomography (CT), and MRI. While the role of dedicated breast PET (dbPET) in BC was initially limited to lesion detection, over the past 2 decades, there has been significant progress in our understanding of how cancer behaves. This includes the ability to categorize BC on the basis hormone receptor status, genetic makeup of cancer cells, and tumor heterogeneity.[10–13] The availability of tumor biology information is thus expected to provide the capability of using dbPET in a number of roles besides lesion detection. While a detailed review of the various clinical applications of dbPET is also separately included in this journal issue, broadly, dbPET can play a role in determining extent of disease in the breast, accurately characterizing tumor biology to influence choice of therapy, treatment planning, and evaluating treatment response prior to and after breast

Department of Radiology, Perelman School of Medicine, University of Pennsylvania, Philadelphia, USA
* Corresponding author.
E-mail address: srilalan@pennmedicine.upenn.edu

PET Clin 19 (2024) 37–47
https://doi.org/10.1016/j.cpet.2023.09.001

conserving surgery. The development of breast cancer-specific radiotracers, including ^{18}F-fluoroestradiol ([18]FES) which recently received Food and Drug Administration (FDA) approval adds to this promise.[14–18]

DEDICATED BREAST PET SCANNERS

Early BC imaging studies which demonstrated the effectiveness of [18]FDG in detecting lesions with very high specificity in a diverse group of patients[19–21] were performed with general purpose whole-body (WB) PET scanners having spatial resolution of more than 5 mm full width at half maximum (FWHM) (eg, reference[22]). While WB-PET scanners provide the ability to image the entire body and find distant metastasis, the cost of a dbPET scanner is much lower than a WB-PET scanner. dbPET scanners also offer lower attenuation as the 511 keV PET photons do not travel through the patient body before reaching the detectors. This will increase the overall scanner sensitivity, lower PET image noise (or scan time), and improve image quality. The biggest limitation of using WB-PET however is the inability to visualize and accurately quantify small (5 mm or smaller in diameter) lesions that are prevalent in early stages of BC. Achieving this with a short scan on a modern WB-PET scanner[23–25] is a very challenging task to accomplish. This has driven the research and development of dbPET scanners.[26] The advances have spanned several areas and include detector development, data acquisition systems, scanner geometry, systems engineering, as well as data and image processing techniques. The following sections review and summarize many of these efforts in order to provide broad overview, current status, and future trends in this area.

Scanners Imaging Compressed Breast with Limited Angular Coverage (Positron Emission Mammography)

As mammography is the most widely used imaging modality for BC, the first generation of dbPET scanners were inspired by mammography and were designed primarily for lesion detection. Positron emission mammography-I (PEM-I) scanner, the first dbPET scanner was developed at the Montreal Neurologial Institute in Canada.[27,28] Unlike WB-PET scanners which use an array of PET detectors arranged in a cylindrical arrangement surrounding the patient, PEM scanners are typically comprised of 2 detector panels around the compressed breast of a seated or standing patient. PEM uses limited-angle image reconstruction for image generation. The PEM-I scanner

made use of a 2-level depth-of-interaction (DOI) detector using layers of finely pixelated bismuth germanate scintillation crystals measuring $1.9 \times 1.9 \times 10$ mm^3 and coupled to position-sensitive photomultiplier (PS-PMT). With an imaging field-of-view (FOV) of 6.5 cm $\times$ 5.5 cm, the PEM scanner was also integrated within a standard mammography unit to provide co-registered images of the breast under compression. Spatial resolution of 2.8 mm FWHM was measured, and DOI helps in maintaining spatial resolution over the imaging FOV. A small pilot study demonstrated that PEM-I scanner could acquire [18]FDG images of diagnostic quality with a short imaging time of 2 to 5 min and still have 80% sensitivity, 100% specificity, and 86% accuracy.[29]

A scanner with identical design concept was also developed shortly thereafter at the National Institute of Health, USA. It utilized a single layer of 10 mm thick bismuth germanium oxide (BGO) crystals to develop a PEM scanner with a 6 cm $\times$ 6 cm imaging FOV. The scanner had spatial resolution of 3.1 mm and also demonstrated the ability to visualize [18]FDG uptake in 1 cm lesions in a ~5 min scan.[30] A collaboration between Duke University and Jefferson Laboratory utilizing $3 \times 3 \times 10$ mm^3 lutetium-gadolinium oxyorthosilicate (LGSO) crystals coupled to a PS-PMT led to the development of a similar scanner design which was integrated with a mammography unit and had spatial resolution of 4.1 mm, and FOV of 15 cm $\times$ 20 cm.[31] A pilot study with this scanner imaging 23 patients with suspected malignancy demonstrated PEMs ability to detect small lesions.[32] A few years later, a group at the University of Texas developed a PEM camera with 20 cm $\times$ 12 cm FOV using $1.5 \times 1.5 \times 10$ mm^3 lutetium-yttrium oxyorthosilicate (LYSO) crystals[33] and a low-cost PMT-quadrant-sharing detector design.[34] Performance characterization of the scanner was presented, but clinical evaluation has not been reported. These first generation of PEM scanners demonstrated the advantages of higher spatial resolution and sensitivity from using PEM for detecting small lesions. Due to limited clinical applications however, it was not widely adopted.

The Naviscan Flex Solo II (now, CMR Naviscan[35]) was the first commercially available PEM scanner. The scanner uses PS-PMT-based flat detectors that measure 6 cm $\times$ 16.4 cm and utilize $2 \times 2 \times 13$ mm^3 LYSO crystals.[36] During imaging, both detectors move in unison to scan the FOV along their 6-cm dimension, and provides an imaging FOV of 24 cm $\times$ 16.4 cm. The detectors and compression paddle are mounted onto an upright gantry that has an articulating arm to help obtain craniocaudal and mediolateral views that are typically obtained with a compressed breast during a mammography examination. The scanner has an in-plane resolution of 2.4 mm and uses a maximum likelihood algorithm-based reconstruction to generate 3-dimensional (3-D) images of the breast.[37] Due to limited-angle effects (ie, lack of complete angular coverage of breast), the z-plane resolution is worse and multiple views of the breast are useful for accurate 3-D localization. The scanner is also compatible with a navigator device which is FDA-approved and provides the ability for image guided biopsy using PEM.[38]

Being commercially available, the Flex Solo II PEM scanner has been the most clinically evaluated dbPET scanner and there have been a number of clinical evaluations to support the potential of PEM. For example, validation that PEM offers higher sensitivity for detecting tumors that are smaller than 1 cm[39,40]; with conclusion that despite having similar sensitivity to MRI, PEM offers higher specificity and is valuable in detecting additional malignancy.[41–43] The Flex Solo II has recently been discontinued and is being replaced by the Solo II High Resolution Breast PEM scanner (**Fig. 1**) which is currently under development.

A group at Stanford University began working on a dual-panel PET scanner using multiple layers of scintillation PET detector modules. Each detector uses a 3 × 8 array of 1 × 1 × 3 mm³ lutetium oxyorthosilicate (LSO) crystals, with its long side coupled to position-sensitive avalanche photodiode.[44,45] The detector panels measure 10 cm × 15 cm and is designed to provide 1 mm spatial resolution along with 3 mm DOI resolution. The same group also studied the use of cadmium zinc telluride (CZT), a high-density semiconductor material,[46] to develop a similar scanner with 4 cm thick panels measuring 12 cm × 15 cm.[47] With 3-D position capability, both of these approaches can provide excellent spatial resolution. CZT also offers exquisite energy resolution. These approaches however, require the use of custom low-noise readout electronics at high channel-density, as well as temperature stabilization which is an additional engineering challenge. While prototype detector panels and a partially completed scanner were developed with commercial readout electronics,[48,49] clinical evaluations have not been performed using either system.

Fairly recently, a group at Xidian University integrated a PEM-design scanner with diffuse optical tomography (DOT).[50] The PEM scanner utilized 1.89 × 1.89 × 13 mm³ LYSO crystals coupled to silicon photomultiplier (SiPM) sensors and PET detector panels measuring 21.6 cm × 14.5 cm to develop a scanner with 12 cm panel separation. During imaging the patient is in the prone position, and the breast tissue is mildly compressed by 2 optical plates primarily to improve DOT signal. While combined PET-DOT scanner performance has not been evaluated, PET only [18]FDG imaging from a small pilot study demonstrated the ability to distinguish small lesions with low uptake. In comparison with WB-PET images, dbPET provided images with high contrast and resolution.

Scanners with Stationary or Rotating Detectors for Imaging Uncompressed Breast with Patient in the Prone Position

It is well known that incomplete angular coverage in PET scanner design leads to non-optimal image quality.[51,52] Fully 3-D tomographic reconstruction can provide the best image quality and quantitative imaging capability. Besides lesion detection, accurate quantification can also help with applications related to BC treatment planning and assessing treatment response. Newer design approaches acquired tomographic breast data by incorporating detector panel rotation or using the panels in a non-circular geometry that eliminated effects from limited angular coverage. Unless specified, all of the following scanners described in this section imaged the patient in prone position and with the uncompressed breast hanging in the scanner FOV.

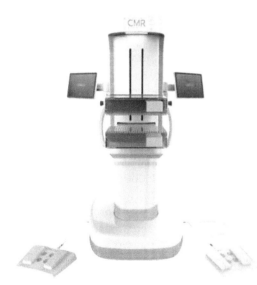

Fig. 1. Photo of the CMR (Companía Mexicana de Radiología) Molecular Imaging (erstwhile Naviscan PET Systems)—Solo II High-Resolution Breast positron emission microscopy (PEM) scanner. This scanner is an updated version of the PEM Flex Solo II scanner that has recently been discontinued. Note that the Solo II High Resolution Breast PEM scanner is under development and currently not available for sale. (Solo II. With permission from CMR Naviscan Corporation.[35])

A team at the University of Pennsylvania developed an early version of breast PET scanner using 2 large, curved plate and NaI(Tl) detectors that were 19 mm thick. The detector panels, each of which measured 28 cm × 21 cm, are placed in a split-ring design on a flexible gantry and can be moved to provide variable detector separation.[53] A pilot [18]FDG imaging study in 20 patients compared images with a contemporary WB-PET scanner and demonstrated good image quality as well as improved detail and contrast.[54]

A team at Lawrence Berkeley National Laboratory developed a box-shaped PEM scanner using their detector modules to provide a rectangular FOV and thereby have complete angular coverage. The detector used 3 × 3 × 30 mm[3] long LSO crystals coupled to a PMT on 1 side and a silicon photodiode on the other end to obtain DOI information.[55] During imaging, the breast was slightly compressed and inserted into the scanner. The distance between the top and bottom detector panels was adjustable to accommodate different breast sizes. Phantom measurements have been presented, but clinical evaluations have not been performed.

A Portuguese PET Mammography consortium within the Crystal Clear Collaboration at *Conseil européen pour la Recherche nucléaire* developed the Clear-PEM scanner.[56] The scanner used 2 × 2 × 10 mm[3] LYSO crystals coupled to an avalanche photodiode (APD) array on both sides of the crystal to enable DOI measurement. The 2 PET detector panels, each measuring 16.5 cm × 14.5 cm were rotated around the scanner axis to collect data at several angular positions necessary for tomographic reconstruction. Instead of a compression-free hanging breast, the breast is encompassed by a cone applying minimal compression. Scanner performance using phantoms and [18]FDG imaging from a single patient without BC have been presented to demonstrate the intrinsic capability of the ClearPEM scanner.

A group at the University of West Virginia[57] also developed a similar system incorporating rotating detector panels. Each detector panel measured 15 cm × 20 cm and used 2 × 2 × 15 mm[3] LYSO crystals readout by a flat panel PMT. A biopsy machine was integrated with the PET scanner in order to utilize PET imaging for verifying needle positioning before tissue sampling. While no breast compression is necessary during imaging, the scanner included a holder to immobilize the breast during imaging. The scanner was used in a pilot study which demonstrated the capability of the scanner to generate good quality images and identify lesions not visible in standard mammograms.[58]

The group at UC Davis developed a dbPET scanner by integrating a PET scanner with detector rotation along with a 768-slice cone-beam CT.[59] The PET panels measured 11.9 cm × 11.9 cm and utilized 3 × 3 × 20 mm[3] LYSO crystals readout by a PS-PMT. The PET panel separation was variable in order to optimize the image acquisition and tomographic image quality based on subject breast size. Custom scanner data corrections to produce quantitative images were developed.[60] A pilot study which imaged 4 patients successfully demonstrated ability to accurately show size, extent, and location of BC. The study from UC Davis also raised the issue of patient motion disrupting PET-CT co-registration when imaging an uncompressed breast. Based on their initial imaging experience, the UC Davis team has planned on upgrading detector and electronics on the PET component of their scanner.[61] The team at the University of West Virginia also subsequently incorporated a CT with their PET scanner described earlier.[62]

A team at Washington University used the virtual pinhole PET concept[63] to develop a PET insert panel that can be placed close to the breast while the patient is being imaged in a WB-PET scanner and lays in the supine position with an uncompressed breast. While the insert by itself does not collect PEM-like data, the insert is used to augment the spatial resolution and sensitivity by collecting additional data between the insert and WB-PET scanner. A couple of prototype inserts were developed to demonstrate local improvements in image resolution and contrast using phantom evaluations.[64,65] The same team at Washington University has also performed simulations to investigate the potential benefits from using a stadium PET scanner geometry combined with additional detector panels on the anterior, posterior sides of the patient. Such a scanner geometry nearly completely surrounds the breast and will provide a larger imaging FOV than currently possible with dbPET.[66]

Full Ring Dedicated Breast-PET Scanners for Imaging Uncompressed Breast in Prone Position

University of Texas developed HOTPET, a high-resolution full-ring PET scanner, using 2.7 × 2.7 × 18 mm[3] BGO crystals.[67] The scanner had a transformable gantry and could be configured into either a WB-PET scanner or brain/breast/axilla PET scanner with 54 cm ring diameter and 21 cm axial FOV. No clinical evaluations were performed, but phantom evaluations demonstrated ability to detect less than or equal to 5 mm lesions with lesion to background contrast of 3.5, not possible with WB-PET available at that time.[68]

A team at Brookhaven National Laboratory developed a prototype full-ring PET insert that was integrated within the radiofrequency coil of an MR scanner. The scanner utilized $2 \times 2 \times 15$ mm^3 LYSO crystals directly coupled to an APD array.[69] A pilot study imaging 4 patients using the PET scanner integrated within a commercial dedicated breast-MR scanner showed good quantitative correlation between PET and MR.[70]

The MAMmography with Molecular Imaging (MAMMI) is a full-ring dbPET scanner (**Fig. 2**) currently commercialized by Oncovision (Valencia, Spain). The scanner uses 10 mm thick monolithic LYSO scintillator coupled to a PS-PMT and provides DOI measurement. The scanner has a transaxial FOV of 17 cm and axial FOV of 4 cm which can be translated to cover up to 17 cm axial length. Spatial resolution of less than 2 mm is measured in the central scanner FOV.[71,72] Scan time for a single ring position takes up to 5 mins, and the total scan time is dependent on the breast size. The scanner has received regulatory approval in both Europe and the United States of America. Koolen and colleagues,[73] performed a first validation of the scanner in 32 patients with invasive BC. Koolen and colleagues,[74] also compared MAMMI with WB-PET to demonstrate the advantage in detecting less than 1 cm lesions as well as discern intra-tumoral heterogeneity. **Figs. 3** and **4** show images from [18]FES imaging study in estrogen receptor positive(ER) + BC which used the MAMMI dbPET scanner for imaging.[75]

Shimadzu (Kyoto, Japan) has commercialized the Elmammo scanner (**Fig. 5**). The scanner uses 4 layers of $1.4 \times 1.4 \times 4.5$ mm^3 LGSO crystals coupled to a PS-PMT. Three rings of 12 detectors

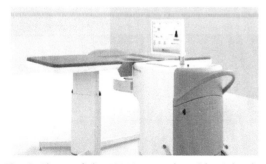

Fig. 2. Photo of the MAMmography with Molecular Imaging (MAMMI PET) scanner. The patient is imaged in the prone position with the breast hanging through an opening in the bed. The PET scanner has an axial field of view (FOV) of 4 cm and can be translated to cover up to 17 cm axial length. (MAMMI PET scanner. With permission from Oncovision.[76])

provide 18 cm FOV and 15.5 cm axial coverage.[78] This scanner has a spatial resolution of less than 2 mm. More recently, they have also developed a variant of this scanner by removing a few detector blocks to convert the full-ring scanner to a C-shaped scanner. Instead of imaging the subject in the prone position, the C-shaped scanner is designed to image with the subject leaning forward. The C-shaped ring also rotates to accommodate the arm based on right or left breast imaging.[79]

Nishimatsu and colleagues[80] compared dbPET images from Elmammo with WB-PET from 179 histologically proven BC lesions in 150 females and categorized them based on size and clinical stage of cancer. As large lesions were not excluded (mean size of 2.59 cm for invasive carcinoma and 1.98 cm for noninvasive carcinoma), it was not surprising that the improvement in sensitivity was not statistically significant. However, dbPET images were more conspicuous and with larger tumor-to-background ratio (suggesting higher contrast recovery) as expected from using dbPET. The Elmammo scanner has received regulatory approval in Japan and China, and consequently several recent investigations have been performed with this device; for example,[81] to determine utility of the scanner in detecting sub-cm and low-grade BC[82]; evaluate its detection rate for ductal carcinoma in situ[83]; investigate its usefulness in classifying BC. Based on the success of the scanner, Shimadzu has also recently commercialized Brestome, a breast/brain reconfigurable time-of-flight (TOF) PET scanner using SiPM and $2.1 \times 2.1 \times 15$ mm^3 LGSO crystal.[84]

Researchers at the Institute of High Energy Physics in China developed PEMi, a polygonal full-ring scanner using 16 modules of detectors employing $1.9 \times 1.9 \times 15$ mm^3 LYSO crystals coupled to PS-PMT.[85] The scanner has a transaxial FOV of 11 cm, axial length of 12.8 cm. A pilot study using [18]FDG in patients with confirmed malignancy was performed using a 15 min scan, and demonstrated good correlation with mammography, as well as the ability to visualize small lesions not seen by WB-PET.

Prescient Medical Imaging recently received FDA clearance for BBX-PET, their portable point-of-care PET scanner.[86] With a flexible gantry, and 25 cm diameter scanner bore and 10 cm axial coverage, the scanner is designed to image breast, brain, and extremities. The scanner utilizes LYSO crystals in a 2-layer DOI design and with a cross-section of 1.7×1.7 mm that is coupled to SiPM. The scanner is advertised to have spatial resolution of 2.2 mm, and performance characterization of the scanner is forthcoming.

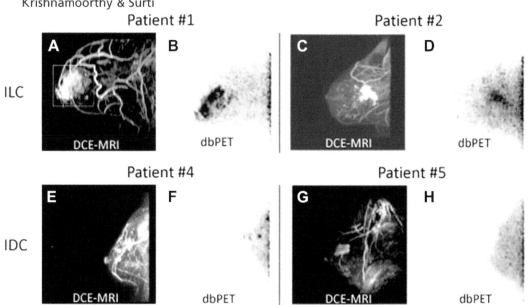

Fig. 3. An example of ^{18}FES uptake from a pilot study using the MAMMI dbPET scanner for 2 categories of BC subjects—Invasive Lobular Carcinoma (ILC) on the top panel (figures A-D), and invasive ductal carcinoma (IDC, bottom panel - figures E-H). Dynamic contrast-enhanced MRI (DCE-MRI) and corresponding dbPET images for 4 patients are shown for each of the 4 subjects. All 4 subjects presented contrast enhancement in their MRI scan, and high SUV$_{max}$ in their corresponding ^{18}FES-dbPET scan. Patient #5 had a recent administration of Tamoxifen, which is an estrogen receptor blocker, and consequently shows no ^{18}FES uptake. (Image reprinted with permission from Jones et al.[75])

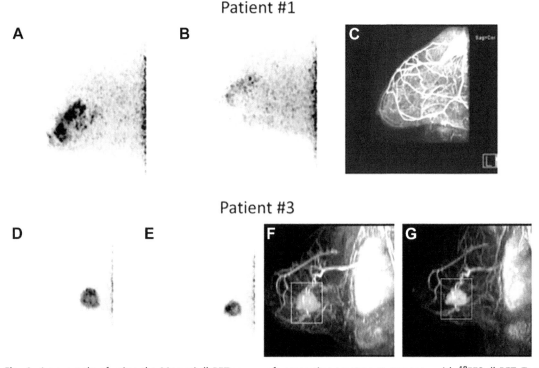

Fig. 4. An example of using the Mammi dbPET scanner for assessing treatment response with ^{18}FES-dbPET. Top: reduction in SUV$_{max}$ observed from dbPET scans in subject with ILC: at baseline (*A*), and 2 months after treatment (*B*). DCE-MRI confirming the favorable response with no residual disease, but significant background enhancement (*C*). Bottom: reduction in SUV$_{max}$ and total uptake volume observed from dbPET scans in subject with IDC: ^{18}FES dbPET scans at baseline (*D*) and post 3-week treatment (*E*). Corresponding DCE MRI (*F*), and (*G*) confirming the tumor size reduction. (Image reprinted with permission from Jones et al.[75])

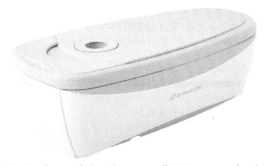

Fig. 5. Photo of the Elmammo dbPET scanner developed by Shimadzu. The PET scanner and patient bed are integrated on a single gantry and the breast is imaged with the subject in the prone position. (Shimadzu - Elmammo - Dedicated Breast PET system. With permission from Shimadzu Corporation.[77])

Ongoing Efforts and Challenges

The last decade has seen tremendous improvements in TOF-PET and is now routinely available in the clinic.[87,88] More recent efforts in developing dbPET scanners include leveraging TOF for dbPET and on improving the quantitation capabilities of the scanner.

Our group at the University of Pennsylvania has developed a TOF-capable dbPET scanner using a PEM-like scanner design for imaging a compressed breast while the patient is seated or standing. The scanner has detector panels measuring 20 cm × 10 cm, and uses $1.5 \times 1.5 \times 15$ mm^3 LYSO crystals readout by a multi-anode PMT. The system is designed to have less than 2 mm spatial resolution and TOF resolution of ~400 ps.[89–91] In such a scanner design, TOF of 300 to 600 ps has shown to alleviate limited-angle artifacts and helps in maintaining quantitative capability.[92] This dbPET scanner has also been integrated with a DBT scanner to provide intrinsically co-registered PET and DBT images. A pilot imaging study using [18]FES radiotracer under an approved institutional review board protocol will open shortly with a goal of evaluating local extent of disease in ER + patients with early-stage BC. A similar approach to build dbPET integrated with mammography was also proposed by a team at the University of Washington.[93–95]

Finally, a collaboration led by a group at Aachen University is developing a PET-insert that will be integrated with a clinical 1.5 T MRI for dbPET-MR imaging. The scanner is expected to have DOI and TOF capability to provide high spatial resolution and sensitivity.[96]

Besides advances in instrumentation and scanner design, we have also witnessed advances in the software realm for dbPET; most notable in the use of deep learning or artificial intelligence (AI). Currently AI is being evaluated on numerous fronts: from detector signal processing to image acquisition, data corrections, and image generation, processing.[97–99] While most of the above are likely to benefit PET in general, the most significant impact in BC is likely in the field of radiomics[100] where we already have seen some preliminary indications.[101–103] As radiomics relies on deriving feature maps (eg, tumor heterogeneity) from imaging data, advances in both hardware and software are relevant for realizing its potential. Among dbPET instrumentation challenges, the ability to image near the edge of the FOV that is particularly close to the chest-wall and axilla is important.

SUMMARY

This review succinctly describes a number of efforts that have advanced the design, development, and imaging performance of dbPET scanners. Until the past decade the efforts were largely academic. A few commercial options with spatial resolution in the 1.5 to 2 mm range, and the ability to provide tomographic, and quantitative data are now available. Hopefully the recent advances in dbPET coupled with the availability of newer breast-specific radiotracers can help continue this momentum and result in larger trials to confirm its potential and possibly increased clinical adoption.

ACKNOWLEDGMENTS

The work was supported in part by NIH grants R01-CA196528, R01-CA113941 and R01-EB028764.

REFERENCES

1. Sung H, Ferlay J, Siegel RL, et al. Global cancer statistics 2020: GLOBOCAN estimates of incidence and mortality worldwide for 36 cancers in 185 countries. CA A Cancer J Clin 2021;71(3):209–49.
2. American Cancer Society - Breast Cancer. cited 2023 March 31; Available from: https://www.cancer.org/cancer/breast-cancer.html.
3. Neal RD, Tharmanathan P, France B, et al. Is increased time to diagnosis and treatment in symptomatic cancer associated with poorer outcomes? Systematic review. Br J Cancer 2015;112(1):S92–107.
4. Chong A, Weinstein SP, McDonald ES, et al. Digital breast tomosynthesis: concepts and clinical practice. Radiology 2019;292(1):1–14.
5. Hooley RJ, Durand MA, Philpotts LE. Advances in digital breast tomosynthesis. Am J Roentgenol 2017;208(2):256–66.

6. Ho T-QH, Bissell MCS, Kerlikowske K, et al. Cumulative probability of false-positive results after 10 years of screening with digital breast tomosynthesis vs digital mammography. JAMA Netw Open 2022;5(3):e222440.

7. Harms of Breast Cancer Screening. Systematic review to update the 2009 u.s. preventive services task force recommendation. Ann Intern Med 2016;164(4):256–67.

8. Iranmakani, S., et al., A review of various modalities in breast imaging: technical aspects and clinical outcomes. 2020. 51(1): p. 57.

9. Catalano O, Fusco R, De Muzio F, et al. Recent advances in ultrasound breast imaging: from industry to clinical practice. Diagnostics 2023;13(5).

10. Dunnwald LK, Rossing MA, Li CI. Hormone receptor status, tumor characteristics, and prognosis: a prospective cohort of breast cancer patients. Breast Cancer Res 2007;9(1):R6.

11. Prat A, Perou CM. Deconstructing the molecular portraits of breast cancer. Mol Oncol 2011;5(1):5–23.

12. Ellis MJ, Perou CM. The genomic landscape of breast cancer as a therapeutic roadmap. Cancer Discov 2013;3(1):27–34.

13. de Mooij CM, Ploumen RAW, Nelemans PJ, et al. The influence of receptor expression and clinical subtypes on baseline [18F]FDG uptake in breast cancer: systematic review and meta-analysis. EJNMMI Res 2023;13(1):5.

14. Linden HM, Dehdashti F. Novel methods and tracers for breast cancer imaging. Semin Nucl Med 2013;43(4):324–9.

15. O'Brien SR, Edmonds CE, Katz D, et al. 18F-Fluoroestradiol (FES) PET/CT: review of current practice and future directions. Clinical and Translational Imaging 2022;10(4):331–41.

16. Hunter N, Peterson L, Mankoff DA, et al. Matched FES and FDG PET imaging in patients with hormone receptor-positive, HER2+ advanced breast cancer. J Clin Oncol 2022;40(16_suppl):1042.

17. Balma M, Liberini V, Racca M, et al. Non-conventional and investigational PET radiotracers for breast cancer: a systematic review. Front Med 2022;9:881551.

18. Cerianna - Fluoroestradiol F18 injection - User Guide. cited 2023 March 31; Available from: https://www.cerianna.com/wp-content/uploads/2020/07/Cerianna-users-guide.pdf.

19. Wahl RL, Cody RL, Hutchins GD, et al. Primary and metastatic breast carcinoma: initial clinical evaluation with PET with the radiolabeled glucose analogue 2-[F-18]-fluoro-2-deoxy-D-glucose. Radiology 1991;179(3):765–70.

20. Adler LP, Crowe JP, al-Kaisi NK, et al. Evaluation of breast masses and axillary lymph nodes with [F-18] 2-deoxy-2-fluoro-D-glucose PET. Radiology 1993;187(3):743–50.

21. Crowe JP Jr, Adler LP, Shenk RR, et al. Positron emission tomography and breast masses: comparison with clinical, mammographic, and pathological findings. Ann Surg Oncol 1994;1(2):132–40.

22. Lewellen TK, Bice A, Harrison R, et al. Performance measurements of the SP3000/UW time-of-flight positron emission tomograph. IEEE Trans Nucl Sci 1988;35(1):665–9.

23. Surti S, Kuhn A, Werner ME, et al. Performance of Philips Gemini TF PET/CT scanner with special consideration for its time-of-flight imaging capabilities. J Nucl Med 2007;48(3):471–80.

24. Jakoby BW, Bercier Y, Conti M, et al. Physical and clinical performance of the mCT time-of-flight PET/CT scanner. Phys Med Biol 2011; 56(8):2375–89.

25. Bettinardi V, Presotto L, Rapisarda E, et al. Physical performance of the new hybrid PET/CT discovery-690. Med Phys 2011;38(10):5394–411.

26. NEMA standards publication NU 2. In: Performance measurements of positron emission tomographs. Washington, DC: National Electrical Manufacturers Association; 1994.

27. Thompson CJ, Murthy K, Picard Y, et al. Positron emission mammography (PEM) - a promising technique for detecting breast-cancer. IEEE Trans Nucl Sci 1995;42(4):1012–7.

28. Thompson CJ, Murthy K, Weinberg IN, et al. Feasibility study for positron emission mammography. Med Phys 1994;21(4):529–38.

29. Murthy K, Aznar M, Thompson CJ, et al. Results of preliminary clinical trials of the positron emission mammography system PEM-I: a dedicated breast imaging system producing glucose metabolic images using FDG. J Nucl Med 2000;41(11):1851.

30. Weinberg I, Majewski S, Weisenberger A, et al. Preliminary results for positron emission mammography: real-time functional breast imaging in a conventional mammography gantry. Eur J Nucl Med 1996;23(7):804–6.

31. Turkington TG, et al. A large field of view positron emission mammography imager, 2002 IEEE Nuclear Science Symposium Conference Record, Norfolk, VA, USA, 2002, pp. 1883–1886 vol.3, doi: 10.1109/NSSMIC.2002.1239690.

32. Rosen EL, Turkington TG, Soo MS, et al. Detection of primary breast carcinoma with a dedicated, large-field-of-view FDG PET mammography device: initial experience. Radiology 2005;234(2): 527–34.

33. Zhang Y, Ramirez RA, Li H, et al. The system design, engineering architecture, and preliminary results of a lower-cost high-sensitivity high-resolution positron emission mammography camera. IEEE Trans Nucl Sci 2010;57(1):104–10.

34. Wai-Hoi W, Uribe J, Hicks K, et al. A 2-dimensional detector decoding study on BGO arrays with

quadrant sharing photomultipliers. IEEE Trans Nucl Sci 1994;41(4):1453–7.

35. Compañía Mexicana de Radiología (CMR) Molecular Imaging. cited 2023 April 3; Available at: www.cmr-naviscan.com.

36. MacDonald LR, Edwards J, Lewellen T, et al. Clinical imaging characteristics of the positron emission mammography camera: PEM Flex Solo II. J Nucl Med 2009;50(10):1666–75.

37. Luo W, Anashkin E, Matthews CG. Performance evaluation of a PEM scanner using the NEMA NU 4—2008 small animal PET standards. IEEE Trans Nucl Sci 2010;57(1):94–103.

38. Kalinyak JE, Schilling K, Berg WA, et al. PET-guided breast biopsy. Breast J 2011;17(2):143–51.

39. Tejerina Bernal A, Tejerina Bernal A, Rabadán Doreste F, et al. Breast imaging: how we manage diagnostic technology at a multidisciplinary breast center. Journal of Oncology 2012;2012:213421.

40. Eo JS, Chun IK, Paeng JC, et al. Imaging sensitivity of dedicated positron emission mammography in relation to tumor size. Breast 2012;21(1):66–71.

41. Schilling K, Narayanan D, Kalinyak JE, et al. Positron emission mammography in breast cancer presurgical planning: comparisons with magnetic resonance imaging. Eur J Nucl Med Mol Imag 2011;38(1):23–36.

42. Berg WA, Madsen KS, Schilling K, et al. Comparative effectiveness of positron emission mammography and MRI in the contralateral breast of women with newly diagnosed breast cancer. AJR Am J Roentgenol 2012;198(1):219–32.

43. Berg WA, Madsen KS, Schilling K, et al. Breast cancer: comparative effectiveness of positron emission mammography and mr imaging in presurgical planning for the ipsilateral breast. Radiology 2011;258(1):59–72.

44. Zhang J, Olcott PD, Chinn G, et al. Study of the performance of a novel 1 mm resolution dual-panel PET camera design dedicated to breast cancer imaging using Monte Carlo simulation. Med Phys 2007;34(2):680–702.

45. Vandenbroucke A, et al. First measurements of a 512 PSAPD prototype of a sub-mm resolution clinical PET camera, 2013 IEEE Nuclear Science Symposium and Medical Imaging Conference (2013 NSS/MIC), Seoul, Korea (South), 2013, pp. 1–4, doi:10.1109/NSSMIC.2013.6829406.

46. Vaska P, et al. Studies of CZT for PET applications, IEEE Nuclear Science Symposium Conference Record, 2005, Fajardo, PR, USA, 2005, pp. 2799-2802, doi: 10.1109/NSSMIC.2005.1596916.

47. Peng H, Levin CS. Design study of a high-resolution breast-dedicated PET system built from cadmium zinc telluride detectors. Phys Med Biol 2010;55(9):2761–88.

48. Hsu DFC, Freese DL, Reynolds PD, et al. Design and performance of a 1 mm3 resolution clinical PET system comprising 3-D position sensitive scintillation detectors. IEEE Trans Med Imag 2018;37(4):1058–66.

49. Abbaszadeh S, Gu Y, Reynolds PD, et al. Characterization of a sub-assembly of 3D position sensitive cadmium zinc telluride detectors and electronics from a sub-millimeter resolution PET system. Phys Med Biol 2016;61(18):6733.

50. Shi Y, Wang Y, Zhou J, et al. DH-Mammo PET: a dual-head positron emission mammography system for breast imaging. Phys Med Biol 2022;67(20):205004.

51. Townsend D, Schorr B, Jeavons A. Three-dimensional image reconstruction for a positron camera with limited angular acceptance. IEEE Trans Nucl Sci 1980;27(1):463–70.

52. Orlov S. Theory of three-dimensional image reconstruction: I Conditions for a complete set of projections. Sov Phys Crystallogr 1976;20:312–4.

53. Freifelder R, Cardi C, Grigoras I, et al. First results of a dedicated breast PET imager, BPET, using NaI(Tl) curve plate detectors, 2001 IEEE Nuclear Science Symposium Conference Record (Cat. No.01CH37310), San Diego, CA, USA, 2001, pp. 1241–1245 vol.3, doi:10.1109/NSSMIC.2001.1008560.

54. Srinivas SM, Greene LR, Currie GM, et al. A dedicated breast positron emission tomography scanner: proof of concept. J Med Imaging Radiat Sci 2014;45(4):435–9.

55. Wang GC, Huber J, Moses W, et al. Characterization of the LBNL PEM camera. Nuclear Science, IEEE Transactions on 2006;53(3):1129–35.

56. Abreu MC, Aguiar J, Almeida F, et al. Design and evaluation of the Clear-PEM scanner for positron emission mammography. Nuclear Science, IEEE Transactions on 2006;53(1):71–7.

57. Raylman RR, Majewski S, Smith MF, et al. The positron emission mammography/tomography breast imaging and biopsy system (PEM/PET): design, construction and phantom-based measurements. Phys Med Biol 2008;53(3):637–53.

58. Raylman RR, Abraham J, Hazard H, et al. Initial clinical test of a breast-PET scanner. J Med Imag Radiation Oncol 2011;55(1):58–64.

59. Bowen SL, Wu Y, Chaudhari AJ, et al. Initial characterization of a dedicated breast PET/CT scanner during human imaging. J Nucl Med 2009;50(9):1401–8.

60. Bowen SL, Ferrero A, Badawi RD. Quantification with a dedicated breast PET/CT scanner. Med Phys 2012;39:2694–707.

61. Ferrero A, Peng Q, Burkett GW, et al. Preliminary performance characterization of DbPET2.1, a PET scanner dedicated to the imaging of the breast and extremities. Biomedical Physics & Engineering Express 2015;1(1):015202.

62. Raylman RR, Van Kampen W, Stolin AV, et al. A dedicated breast-PET/CT scanner: evaluation of

basic performance characteristics. Med Phys 2018;45(4):1603–13.

63. Yuan-Chuan T, Wu H, Pal D, et al. Virtual-pinhole PET. J Nucl Med 2008;49(3):471.

64. Mathews AJ, Komarov S, Kume MH. et al. Investigation of breast cancer detectability using PET insert with whole-body and zoom-in imaging capability, 2011 IEEE International Symposium on Biomedical Imaging: From Nano to Macro, Chicago, IL, USA, 2011, pp. 1784–1787, doi:10.1109/ISBI.2011.5872752.

65. Ravindranath B, Wei J, Matthews A, et al. A flat panel virtual-pinhole PET insert for axillary and internal mammary lymph node imaging in breast cancer patients. J Nucl Med Meeting Abstract 2012;53:432.

66. Samanta S, Jiang J, Hamdi M, et al. Performance comparison of a dedicated total breast PET system with a clinical whole-body PET system: a simulation study. Phys Med Biol 2021;66(11).

67. Li H, Wong WH, Baghaei H, et al. The engineering and initial results of a transformable low-cost high-resolution PET camera. IEEE Trans Nucl Sci 2007; 54(5):1583–8.

68. Baghaei H, Li H, Zhang Y, et al. A breast phantom lesion study with the high resolution transformable HOTPET camera. IEEE Trans Nucl Sci 2010;57(5):2504–9.

69. Ravindranath B, et al. Results from prototype II of the BNL simultaneous PET-MRI dedicated breast scanner, 2009 IEEE Nuclear Science Symposium Conference Record (NSS/MIC), Orlando, FL, USA, 2009, pp. 3315–3317, doi:10.1109/NSSMIC.2009.5401742.

70. Ravindranath B, Huang P, Junnarkar S, et al. Quantitative clinical evaluation of a simultaneous PET/MRI breast imaging system. J Nucl Med 2012; 53(supplement 1):1217.

71. Moliner L, Gonzalez AJ, Soriano A, et al. Design and evaluation of the MAMMI dedicated breast PET. Med Phys 2012;39(9):5393.

72. García Hernández T, Vicedo González A, Ferrer Rebolleda J, et al. Performance evaluation of a high resolution dedicated breast PET scanner. Med Phys 2016;43(5):2261–72.

73. Koolen BB, Aukema TS, González Martínez AJ, et al. First clinical experience with a dedicated PET for hanging breast molecular imaging. Q J Nucl Med Mol Imaging 2013;57(1):92–100.

74. Koolen BB, Vidal-Sicart S, Benlloch Baviera JM, et al. Evaluating heterogeneity of primary tumor (18)F-FDG uptake in breast cancer with a dedicated breast PET (MAMMI): a feasibility study based on correlation with PET/CT. Nucl Med Commun 2014;35(5):446–52.

75. Jones EF, Ray KM, Li W, et al. Initial experience of dedicated breast PET imaging of ER+ breast cancers using [F-18]fluoroestradiol. NPJ Breast Cancer 2019;5(12).

76. ONCOVISION - MAMMI PET scanner. cited 2023 July 31; Available from: https://oncovision.com/mammi-project/.

77. Shimadzu - Elmammo - Dedicated Breast PET system. cited 2023 April 3; Available from: https://www.shimadzu.com/med/sites/shimadzu.com.med/files/products/pet-imaging/elmammo/ac19-0021_elmammo.pdf.

78. Miyake KK, Matsumoto K, Inoue M, et al. Performance evaluation of a new dedicated breast PET scanner using NEMA NU4-2008 standards. J Nucl Med 2014;55(7):1198–203.

79. Iima M, Nakamoto Y, Kanao S, et al. Clinical performance of 2 dedicated PET scanners for breast imaging: initial evaluation. J Nucl Med 2012;53: 1534–42.

80. Nishimatsu K, Nakamoto Y, Miyake KK, et al. Higher breast cancer conspicuity on dbPET compared to WB-PET/CT. Eur J Radiol 2017;90:138–45.

81. Sueoka S, Sasada S, Masumoto N, et al. Performance of dedicated breast positron emission tomography in the detection of small and low-grade breast cancer. Breast Cancer Res Treat 2021; 187(1):125–33.

82. Masumoto N, Kadoya T, Fujiwara M, et al. Dedicated breast PET to improve clinical diagnosis of breast cancer: initial evaluation. J Clin Oncol 2017;35(15_suppl):e12097.

83. Shinsuke S, Masumoto N, Kimura Y, et al. Classification of abnormal findings on ring-type dedicated breast PET for the detection of breast cancer. Anticancer Res 2020;40(6):3491.

84. Morimoto-Ishikawa D, Hanaoka K, Watanabe S, et al. Evaluation of the performance of a high-resolution time-of-flight PET system dedicated to the head and breast according to NEMA NU 2-2012 standard. EJNMMI Physics 2022;9(1):88.

85. Li L, Gu XY, Li DW, et al. Performance evaluation and initial clinical test of the positron emission mammography system (PEMi). IEEE Trans Nucl Sci 2015;62(5):2048–56.

86. Prescient Medical Imaging - BBX-PET. cited 2023 April 7; Available from: http://prescient-imaging.com/products/.

87. Surti S, Karp JS. Advances in time-of-flight PET. Phys Med: European Journal of Medical Physics 2016;32(1):12–22.

88. Schaart DR. Physics and technology of time-of-flight PET detectors. Phys Med Biol 2021;66(9):09TR01.

89. Krishnamoorthy S, Vent T, Barufaldi B, et al. Evaluating attenuation correction strategies in a dedicated, single-gantry breast PET-tomosynthesis scanner. Phys Med Biol 2020;65(23):235028.

90. Krishnamoorthy S, Morales E, Ashmanskas WJ, et al. Performance of PET imaging in a dedicated breast PET-DBT scanner. J Nucl Med 2021; 62(supplement 1):1145.

91. Krishnamoorthy S, Morales E, Ashmanskas WJ, et al. Imaging performance of a dedicated BPET-DBT scanner. J Nucl Med 2022;63(supplement 2): 2439.

92. Surti S, Karp JS. Design considerations for a limited angle, dedicated breast, TOF PET scanner. Phys Med Biol 2008;53(11):2911–21.

93. MacDonald LR, Hunter WCJ, Kinahan PE, et al. Effects of detector thickness on geometric sensitivity and event positioning errors in the rectangular PET/X scanner. IEEE Trans Nucl Sci 2013;60(5): 3242–52.

94. MacDonald, LR, Hunter WCJ, Zeng C, et al. The PET/X dedicated breast-PET scanner for optimizing cancer therapy, Proc. SPIE 10718, 14th International Workshop on Breast Imaging (IWBI 2018), 107180M (6 July 2018); https://doi.org/10.1117/12. 2318419.

95. MacDonald LR, Lo JY, Sturgeon GM, et al. Impact of using uniform attenuation coefficients for heterogeneously dense breasts in a dedicated breast PET/X-Ray scanner. IEEE Transactions on Radiation and Plasma Medical Sciences 2020;4:585–93.

96. Schulz V, Weissler B, Nadig V, et al. A dedicated PET insert for a 1.5T MR system for simultaneous breast PET/MRI. Nuklearmedizin 2021;60(02):L17.

97. Reader AJ, Corda G, Mehranian A, et al. Deep learning for PET image reconstruction. IEEE Transactions on Radiation and Plasma Medical Sciences 2021;5(1):1–25.

98. Visvikis D, Lambin P, Beuschau Mauridsen K, et al. Application of artificial intelligence in nuclear medicine and molecular imaging: a review of current status and future perspectives for clinical translation. Eur J Nucl Med Mol Imaging 2022;49(13): 4452–63.

99. Saboury B, Bradshaw T, Boellaard R, et al. Artificial intelligence in nuclear medicine: opportunities, challenges, and responsibilities toward a trustworthy ecosystem. J Nucl Med 2023;64(2):188–96.

100. Lambin P, Leijenaar RTH, Deist TM, et al. Radiomics: the bridge between medical imaging and personalized medicine. Nat Rev Clin Oncol 2017; 14(12):749–62.

101. Urso L, Manco L, Castello A, et al. PET-derived radiomics and artificial intelligence in breast cancer: a systematic review. Int J Mol Sci 2022;23(21).

102. Aide N, Salomon T, Blanc-Fournier C, et al. Implications of reconstruction protocol for histo-biological characterisation of breast cancers using FDG-PET radiomics. EJNMMI Res 2018;8.

103. Park H, Lim Y, Ko ES, et al. Radiomics signature on magnetic resonance imaging: association with disease-free survival in patients with invasive breast cancer. Clin Cancer Res 2018;24(19):4705–14.

Developments in Dedicated Prostate PET Instrumentation

Antonio J. Gonzalez, PhD*, Andrea Gonzalez-Montoro, PhD

KEYWORDS

- Positron emission tomography (PET) • Organ-dedicated PET • Prostate cancer (PCa)
- Prostate-specific membrane antigen (PSMA) • Transrectal PET probe

KEY POINTS

- Organ-dedicated PET may help improving early diagnose and staging of prostate cancer (PCa).
- Transrectal PET probes may enable guided biopsies of the prostate and thus, enhance PCa diagnosis.
- New PET instrumentation has to promote sensitivity and homogeneous 3D spatial resolutions of 1 to 2 mm.
- Despite its benefits, there are no commercial PET systems dedicated to the prostate. Further improvements in instrumentation are required to introduce them in the market.

INTRODUCTION

Prostate cancer (PCa) constitutes one of the major health problems facing the male population, being the second most common cause of cancer death in men with an estimated 1.4 million new diagnoses worldwide.[1]

The incidence of PCa is more pronounced between different geographic areas. For example, in Western and Northern Europe, PCa is the most common form of cancer in men, with age standardized rates (ASR) per 100,000 of 94.9 and 85.0, respectively. Although ASR in Eastern and Southern Europe are lower, they have grown.[2,3] Indeed, since 1985, the number of deaths from PCa has increased even in countries or regions where PCa is not common.[4] PCa is more frequent in developed countries where the proportion of elderly men is large with a prevalence of 59% (48%–71%) by age greater than 79 years.[5] However, its impact on male mortality (3% of deaths) is relatively small compared with other cancers, but it may worsen in view of the aging of the population. Thus, PCa is not always considered clinically significant, meaning that it may not cause morbidity or death.

Clinical Diagnose of Prostate Cancer

It is critical to diagnose PCa as soon as possible since the cancer stage at the moment of its identification dictates the prognosis of the patient. PCa is usually suspected during digital rectal examinations (DREs) and/or the identification of abnormal prostate-specific antigen (PSA) levels. Definitive diagnosis depends on histopathological verification of adenocarcinoma in prostate biopsy cores. In the following sections, the main PCa diagnostic methods, which are used complementarily, are described and shown in **Fig. 1**.

Digital rectal examination

Approximately 18% of confirmed PCa cases are first detected by abnormal DRE which is usually associated with an increased risk of a higher grade PCa and is used as an indication for MRI and biopsy.[6,7]

Instituto de Instrumentación para Imagen Molecular (I3M), Centro Mixto CSIC - Universitat Politècnica de València, Camino de Vera s/n, E-46022 Valencia, Spain
* Corresponding author. Instituto de Instrumentacion para Imagen Molecular (i3M), Ciudad Politecnica de la Innovacion, Edif. 8B Acceso N planta 1, Camino de Vera s/n, Valencia 46022, Spain.
E-mail address: agonzalez@i3m.upv.es

PET Clin 19 (2024) 49–57
https://doi.org/10.1016/j.cpet.2023.06.001
1556-8598/24/© 2023 Elsevier Inc. All rights reserved.

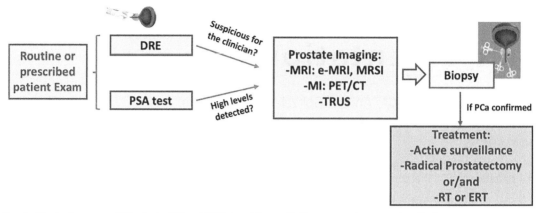

Fig. 1. Block diagram of PCa tests. RT and ERT stand for radiotherapy and external radiotherapy.

Prostate-specific antigen

Serum PSA levels increase with advancing PCa stage. Nevertheless, since PSA is produced by both benign and malignant prostatic tissue, there is no direct relationship between PSA concentration and the clinical and pathologic tumor stage.[8] However, in general, patients with PSA levels below 0.09 ng/mL/cc were found unlikely (4%) to be diagnosed with clinically significant PCa.[9]

Blood and urine biomarkers

Different biomarkers such as the ones detectable in the blood (eg, thrombospondin-1, cathepsin-D) or in urine (eg, PCA3, ERG) are good indicators of PCa especially in the case of incorrect MRI interpretation.[10]

Imaging techniques

Despite less than 60% of tumors are visible with TransRectal UltraSound (TRUS),[11] this technique constitutes the most common method for imaging the prostate. Yet, endorectal MRI (e-MRI) may allow for more accurate local staging[12] since image quality and localization improves significantly compared with external coil MRI.[13] MR spectroscopic imaging (MRSI) assesses tumor metabolism by displaying the relative concentrations of chemical metabolites such as choline, with the potential for a non-invasive assessment of PCa aggressiveness.[14] Unfortunately, e-MRI and MRSI present limitations such as difficulties in interpreting changes of the prostate, and the significant variability among radiologists.

Biopsy

The decision of biopsy is based on a combination of the measured levels of PSA, other biomarkers, suspicious DRE, and/or doubtful imaging. Age, potential co-morbidity, and therapeutic consequences are also considered.[15] During prostate biopsy several tissue cores are randomly taken from the prostate. However, biopsy samplings cover a minuscule part of the prostate, making it easy to omit regions where cancerous cells may lurk. Moreover, the procedure is not painless and may cause infection, fever, bleeding, and other conditions requiring hospitalization. Overall, and despite screening programs, only 55% of the tumors are clinically localized at the time of diagnosis. For this reason, it is desirable to develop a noninvasive and precise (more than current MRI or TRUS) imaging technique for biopsy guidance.

Molecular imaging

Molecular imaging (MI) techniques such as PET/computed tomography (CT) are promising tools for early detection, staging, and biopsy guidance of PCa. Three different types of tracers in PET/CT scans are used, namely (i) choline PET/CT, used for lymph node (LN) identification in the pelvic area. However, due to its low sensitivity, it does not reach clinically acceptable diagnostic accuracy.[16] (ii) prostate specific membrane antigen (PSMA) PET/CT is an attractive target due to its specificity for prostatic tissue. Typically, these studies used ^{68}Ga- or ^{18}F-labelling. Note that, ^{68}Ga-PSMA was found to have a higher sensitivity and a comparable specificity than MRI for staging pre-operative LN metastases in intermediate- and high-risk PCa,[17] and (iii) fluoride PET/CT only assesses the presence of bone metastases, but was reported to have superior sensitivity than conventional bone scintigraphy in patients with newly diagnosed high-risk PCa.[18]

According to the guidelines from the European Association of Urology (EAU), despite significant efforts, conventional imaging of PCa does not contribute to patient management as much as imaging does for other common cancers. In addition, these imaging tests yield little information to differentiate aggressive from indolent disease.

Therefore, there is considerable interest in developing specific biomarkers and accurate noninvasive imaging techniques that will ideally quantify aggressiveness, extent, and burden of disease. Encouragingly, and as described in the next sections, recent advances in technology have opened the way for designing and transferring to the clinics PET systems suitable for PCa.

PET PROSTATE IMAGING

To date, there are no commercial prostate dedicated PET systems and therefore, clinical whole-body PET (WB-PET) scanners are used for PCa examinations. However, using standard WB-PET for PCa diagnosis is not optimal, since these clinical systems offer spatial resolution in the range of 4 to 5 mm at the system center,[19] making it difficult to visualize cancerous lesions in the prostate. The spatial resolution requirements for the detection of prostatic lesions are practically the same as for the ones required in animal models (<1 mm) and the ultimate limit is imposed by the specificity of the imaging agents and uptake in the lesions.[20–22]

Promisingly, recent developments of highly specific PET tracers have increased the interest of using PET for PCa diagnosis and staging, which has encouraged researchers to develop detector technology suitable for prostate dedicated PET.

Prostate Dedicated PET Systems

Dedicated PET scanners have demonstrated to provide higher sensitivity than WB-PET since the detectors can be placed closer to the area under study.[23] PET sensitivity is proportional to the angular coverage provided by the scanner; thus, maximum sensitivity is reached when the scanner is in contact with the external surface of the patient, as happens with dedicated systems, and completely surrounding the body. Moreover, since each patient has different size, optimal geometries cannot be achieved with current PET technology. Thus, dedicated PET should provide better image contrast recovery due to reduced noise coming from the surrounding organs.

Regarding other technical specifications, most of the detector designs used in dedicated PET allow reaching spatial resolutions in the range of 1 to 2 mm, while simultaneously enabling time-of-flight (TOF) capabilities. Furthermore, compared with conventional WB-PET, fewer mechanical components are needed; thus, dedicated systems are more affordable. As a drawback, it must be mentioned that dedicated scanners mainly focus on one organ or area, and thus their use is limited.

Focusing on PCa, one of the first attempts to build a dedicated prostate PET system was presented in 2005 by Huber and colleagues.[24] The system geometry defined 2 arcs constructed with about only one-quarter of the detectors of a commercial WB-PET. The distance between the 2 arcs could be adjusted to allow patient of different sizes and to position the detectors as close as possible for optimized sensitivity. Preliminary results demonstrated similar sensitivity and resolution (approximately 4 mm) as what was reported for standard WB-PET at that time; thus, further improvements were required.

Following this approach, a similar concept was recently developed by Cañizares and colleagues[25] with a geometry defined by a ring of 42 cm in diameter, placed on top of a translational stage allowing to axially cover 80 mm. The 2 top quarters of the ring were openable to allow for an easy patient positioning. The detectors were based on 15 mm thick LYSO monolithic blocks coupled to silicon photomultiplier (SiPM) arrays and readout using custom designed analog boards without TOF capabilities. Note that the monolithic design was key to retrieve the 3D photon impact position which included photon depth of interaction (DOI) information. 3D capabilities make it possible to provide almost uniform spatial resolutions across the entire field of view (FOV) of the scanner. This design reached an average full width at half maximum (FWHM) of 2 mm, without significantly degrading toward the edge of the scanner.[25] Tests carried out with phantoms exhibited good performance, improving over that of conventional systems. However, the lack of transmission information or accurate co-registration with existing CT images made it difficult to interpret the results in patients.

To assess the feasibility of a dedicated compact limited angle coverage system, Turkington and colleagues[26] built a dedicated PET prototype using 2 rotating high-resolution (2 mm FWHM) PET panels with 20 × 15 cm² area each. The sensitivity and uniformity of response in 3D were limited as non-TOF information was provided to account for the lack of angular coverage. **Fig. 2** shows examples of dedicated systems.

The main conclusions of these studies were that detection of PET radiotracer uptake in small and deep structures such as the pelvis or the prostate is possible with dedicated detectors, and the image quality is best when angular acceptance is not limited or most likely when TOF capabilities are enabled. Thus, there are still major technological challenges that have to be overcome to construct prostate dedicated-PET. One of the most investigated approaches is combining existing PET scanners with PET probes, as described in the following section.

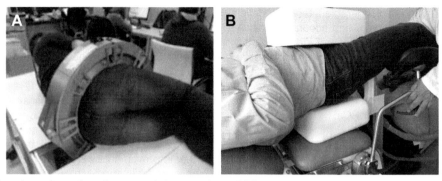

Fig. 2. (*A*) Dedicated ring based on monolithic crystals, and (*B*) Two panels PET prototype built by the authors.

Dedicated-PET Probes

There is a sharp mismatch between the sizes of the cancerous lesions to be detected in the prostate and the resolution of WB-PET and prostate dedicated-PET. Moreover, available detector technology report insufficient sensitivity that imposes long scanning times and reduced patient throughput.

As an alternative to develop new PET scanners, it has been proposed to complement the already existing PET (both clinical and dedicated) with a transrectal PET imaging probe placed close to the prostate, see **Fig. 3** right. Properly combining these tools may improve diagnosis (guided biopsy) and follow-up of patients with PCa. PET-probe systems require specific detector designs, accurate relative positioning of the probe and the scanner, and appropriate image reconstruction algorithms able to combine the different type of coincidences namely scan-scan and scan-probe. The key idea is that by using transrectal PET imaging probes, higher sensitivities will be achieved owing to the proximity of the detector probe–which is usually based on small elements to facilitate insertion as well as to promote high resolution (magnification effect)–to the prostate region, as shown in **Fig. 3**.

One of the first efforts following the concept of magnifying PET was introduced by Huh and colleagues.[22] In this work (based on simulations), a very high resolution detector probe with $1 \times 1 \times 3$ mm^3 LSO crystals was placed close to the organ under study and allowed coincidences with an external PET ring. Therefore, there were 2 types of coincidences (scan-scan and scan-probe). In the scan-scan coincidences, all the detectors had the same spatial resolution while in the scan-probe coincidences the detectors in the probe presented more demanding designs that yielded higher resolution. Therefore, in this second case the reconstructed image of the lesion was magnified allowing to observe small details. Moreover, this approach would help for MI-guided biopsy.

The probe concept has also been experimentally explored. Delfino and colleagues[27] presented a probe detector with DOI capabilities, based on a double-side SiPM readout and $1 \times 1 \times 20$ mm^3 LYSO scintillators. Majewski and colleagues[28]

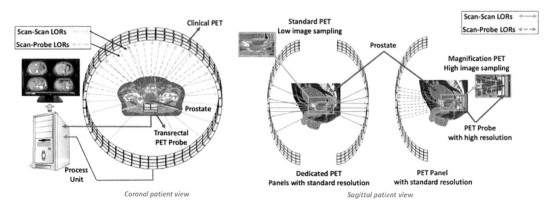

Fig. 3. Left, sketch of a clinical WB-PET + probe. Right, representation of the dedicated (2 panels or arcs) and magnification PET (PET panel + probe) approaches.

designed a dedicated prostate mobile PET system that was implemented in combination with an outside high-resolution PET imager placed close to the patient's torso and an insertable transrectal probe placed in proximity to the prostate. The probe was used in conjunction with the outside imager panel, and the 2 detector systems were spatially co-registered. The outside imager was mounted on an open rotating gantry to provide torso-wide 3D images of the prostate, surrounding tissue and organs. Clinthorne and colleagues[29] reported on a novel concept based on 2 arcs but constructed using BGO scintillators. These arcs were combined with a small silicon detector placed in close proximity to the area under study. Results demonstrated the higher performance achieved when properly merging the scan-scan and the scan-silicon coincidences.

Recently, due to the advances in detector technology and electronics, new probe designs including TOF features have been suggested. Miyaoka and colleagues[30] investigated a probe design for endorectal PET prostate imaging, with high spatial resolution (1 mm) and a temporal precision of 150 ps FWHM. Herein, the probe could be used in coincidence with the external PET or with a detector panel placed over the prostate. More recently, Miyaoka and colleagues[31] also suggested a 2 arcs system (see **Fig. 4**) based on a front detector optimized for CTR performance and a rear detector optimized for 3D positioning and detection efficiency.

Since PCa diagnosis is currently followed by an MRI test, Garibaldi and colleagues[32] introduced the concept of an MRI compatible TOF-PET probe within the TOPEM project. The project aimed at developing a prototype of an endorectal PET-TOF/MRI probe. The expected spatial resolution in the selected geometry was about 1.5 mm FWHM with DOI less than 1 mm and timing resolutions of ~320 ps FWHM.[33]

Similarly, other designs have been proposed using a US probe.[34] It was presented as an improved version of the 2-arcs prostate system (described above) which now included a TRUS probe to help determine the locations of the lesions within the prostate region. It is worth mentioning that in the scope of the funded European Endo-TOFPET project,[35] a prototype PET probe plus PET panel system was designed and built for applications in imaging pancreatic and prostate cancers.

Nevertheless, prostate imaging can be improved not only with dedicated system or PET + probe approaches, but also by increasing the detection capabilities of existing or novel instrumentation. Focused on increasing the sensitivity of clinical systems for PCa, the 2 main paths are as follows.

i. Including TOF information during the image reconstruction process.
ii. Increasing the axial length of the scanner, and thus improving the solid angle coverage by designing total-body PET (TB-PET) with an axial coverage that extends to about 70 cm.[36]

Effects of Time-of-flight Capabilities

In WB-PET, an important milestone was reached when the Siemens Biograph Vision was launched exhibiting a timing resolution of 214 ps FWHM.[37,38] The TOF capabilities showed a significant increase in lesion detectability, especially for those with low uptake or small size.[39] Indeed, one of the most important research topics in PET focuses on improving the coincidence time resolution (CTR) of PET detectors whose limit is mainly imposed by the scintillator, photosensor technology, and associated electronics.

1. Using scintillators with short decay and rise times. The most commonly used scintillators in TOF-PET are lutetium-based, such as

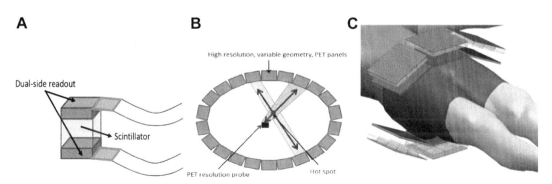

Fig. 4. (*A*) Sketch of a dual PET probe, (*B*) scheme of the probe and PET ring approach and (*C*) 2 arcs PET system with dual layer detectors pixelated and monolithic, respectively.

LYSO, LSO, or LGSO. Recently, it was proposed using crystals with a measurable yield of prompt photons (ie, Cherenkov photons) which are generated much faster than the scintillation ones and thus provide an excellent signature of the arrival time of the event. In this context, BGO may be a promising solution; however, exploiting the low Cherenkov yield imposes challenges related to the photosensor technology and electronics.[40] Other works suggest for instance the concept of meta-scintillators in which dense crystals such as BGO or LYSO are combined with very fast scintillators (plastic or BaF_2).[41]

2. Using enhanced photosensor technology. SiPMs are the preferred option for TOF-PET. The most relevant SiPM parameters affecting CTR are photon detection efficiency (PDE(λ,V)); quantum efficiency (QE(λ)); gain; temperature coefficient; linearity response to the incident radiation; compactness; and time jitter. Recent advancements in SiPM technology present extended PDE and upgraded electric field designs of the single-photon avalanche diode configuration that improve the single photon time response (SPTR) of the detector that dictates the CTR limits.

3. Implementing fast and noiseless electronics to precisely determine the arrival time of the photons. Electronic readout circuits must reduce the device effective capacitance of SiPMs to improve single photon response shape and minimize the influences of noise on the SPTR. Different readout topologies have been proposed, such as the bootstrapping techniques (hardly scalable) or the ones using application specific integrated circuits.[40]

Some studies have already reported on the benefits of using TOF information in PET for the management of PCa. In one of the works the authors implemented a TOF reconstruction for ^{18}F-choline PET/MRI showing higher standard uptake value measurements compared with non-TOF reconstructions.[42] These results also suggested that adding TOF information has a positive impact on lesion detection rate for LN and bone metastasis in patients with PCa. In a separated work, the authors scanned 20 patients and concluded that TOF reconstruction for ^{18}F-choline PET/MR might improve lesion detection rate in patients with PCa.[43]

Total-body PET

TB-PET boosts the physical detection efficiency and, thus, the clinical sensitivity, due to a larger axial coverage.[36,44] Building TB systems imposes major technological challenges such as huge amounts of data to be stored and processed, or fast image reconstruction, among others. Moreover, the higher production cost and complex hardware of long axial PET restrict easy adoption by hospitals and research centers.

The main advantage of using TB-PET for PCa relies on the fact that the higher sensitivity of these scanners helps detecting PCa at the earliest stages (small lesions or low uptake), especially for those with low PSA levels (<30%). In a pilot work an improvement in the detectability rates from patients with biochemically recurrent PCa, and also its impact on therapeutic decisions were demonstrated.[45] TB-PET may also provide enhanced imaging of biomarkers related to intratumor heterogeneity and PET radiomics useful in novel therapy such as theragnostics.[46] **Fig. 5** shows the different PET approaches described in this section, highlighting the main advantages and disadvantages of each one.

It should be mentioned that other ways to extend the use of PET in PCa have been proposed and are based on introducing artificial intelligence

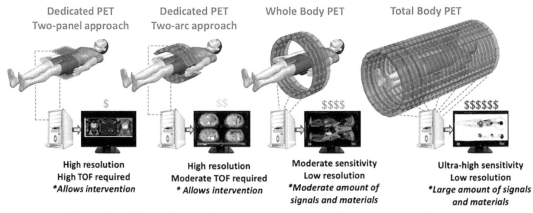

Fig. 5. From left to right, dedicated 2 panels, 2 arcs, WB- and TB-PET designs, respectively.

(AI) techniques at the detector level (to improve the 3D photon interaction positioning) and at system level (to classify and evaluate PET images of the prostate). From the clinical perspectives, AI may provide a deeper understanding of the molecular environment of PCa, refining personalized treatment strategies, and increasing the ability to predict the outcome.[47]

INTERVENTIONAL TECHNIQUES

Interventional techniques could help in PCa detectability and follow-up. HIgh specificity MI agents are used as driving molecules for theragnostic or to drive the chemotherapy agents to PCa specific cells minimizing secondary side effects.

Local (prostatic) injection of the theragnostic or radiotracer compound may optimize treatment by delivering a higher dose at the target (ie, the prostate). Lower dose requirements will make it possible saving in patient and clinicians' risks, but also radiopharmacology costs. By directly injecting the agent in the prostate, it can also be observed the possible derange to the LN with conventional imaging. Dedicated prostate PET scanners could eventually be used in less radiation restrictive area due to the lower dose.

Developments of PET ligands such as ^{18}F-labeled choline analogs, ^{11}C-acetate, ^{68}Ga, ^{18}F-fluorocyclobutane-1-carboxylic acid fluciclovine (FACBC), and ^{18}F-fluorodihydrotestosterone have shown promising results in the detection of malignant lesions in PCa.[48] A more advanced solution is to search for PCa-specific antigenic targets such as PSMA, and generate agents able to specifically bind. Although advances in conventional imaging will continue, antibody and small molecule imaging exemplified by PSMA targeting have the greatest potential to improve diagnostic sensitivity and specificity.[40] There Is a continuous Interest to develop monoclonal antibodies designed to target PSMA[50] and many have shown good results for PET imaging of metastatic PCa.[51]

SUMMARY

Some specific MI designs assessing early detection and staging of PCa have been proposed. It can be differentiated between systems (dedicated-, WB- and TB-PET), and inserts or probes that are placed much closer to the prostate with the aim to boost spatial resolution (magnification effect) and eventually sensitivity in the area under observation. Fully prostate-dedicated systems have not yet reached an optimum of performance to be transferred to the clinics or industry, most

likely due to the lack of precise detectors able to include DOI and TOF capabilities simultaneously at an affordable cost. Moreover, several attempts have been carried out in a variety of probe technologies such as PET alone, US combined, with TOF capabilities and even MRI compatible, reporting promising results.

It seems very likely that using images provided by prostate dedicated-PET scanners for biopsy guidance would help in diagnosis. As reviewed in the present article, this may be accomplished with dedicated prostate PET using for instance TransRectal PET imaging probes resulting in a high sensitivity.

As an alternative to dedicated PET and the combination PET probe, currently available PET scanners could be technologically upgraded by designing more precise detectors or/and by including AI techniques. To accomplish these goals, advancements in the detection technology are required. There have been several encouraging attempts during the last years on these lines, and it seems feasible that enhanced PET and TB-PET technology may become a reality soon, and thus, their use could be extended for PCa.

DISCLOSURE

The authors have nothing to disclose.

FUNDING

We thank financial support from Generalitat Valenciana through the program Equipamiento e Infraestructuras FEDER 2021-22 IDIFEDER/2021/004.

ACKNOWLEDGMENTS

The authors would like to thank S. Majewski for providing hints of some prostate dedicated systems. They would also like to acknowledge the contribution of Dr. Cesar D. Vera Donoso for his proof reading of clinical aspects of this article.

REFERENCES

1. Culp MB, Soerjomataram I, Efstathiou JA, et al. Recent global patterns in prostate cancer incidence and mortality rates. Eur Urol 2020;77(1):38–52.
2. Haas GP, Delongchamps N, Brawley OW, et al. The worldwide epidemiology of prostate cancer: perspectives from autopsy studies. Can J Urol 2008; 15(1):3866–71.
3. Boyle P, Ferlay J. Cancer incidence and mortality in Europe 2004. Ann Oncol 2005;16:481–8.
4. Quinn M, Babb P. Patterns and trends in prostate cancer incidence, survival, prevalence and mortality.

Part I: international comparisons. BJU Int 2002;90:162–73.

5. Bell KJ, Del Mar C, Wright G, et al. Prevalence of incidental prostate cancer: a systematic review of autopsy studies. Int J Cancer 2015;137(7):1749–57.

6. Gosselaar C, Roobol MJ, Roemeling S, et al. The role of the digital rectal examination in subsequent screening visits in the European randomized study of screening for prostate cancer (ERSPC), Rotterdam. Eur Urol 2008;54(3):581–8.

7. Okotie OT, Roehl KA, Han M, et al. Characteristics of prostate cancer detected by digital rectal examination only. Urology 2007;70(6):1117–20.

8. Partin AW, Carter HB, Chan DW, et al. Prostate specific antigen in the staging of localized prostate cancer: influence of tumor differentiation, tumor volume and benign hyperplasia. J Urol 1990;143(4):747–52.

9. Yusim I, Krenawi M, Mazor E, et al. The use of prostate specific antigen density to predict clinically significant prostate cancer. Sci Rep 2020;10(1):20015.

10. Tomlins SA, Rhodes DR, Perner S, et al. Recurrent fusion of TMPRSS2 and ETS transcription factor genes in prostate cancer. Science 2005;310(5748):644–8.

11. Smith JA Jr, Scardino PT, Resnick MI, et al. Transrectal ultrasound versus digital rectal examination for the staging of carcinoma of the prostate: results of a prospective, multi-institutional trial. J Urol 1997;157(3):902–6.

12. Masterson TA, Touijer K. The role of endorectal coil MRI in preoperative staging and decision-making for the treatment of clinically localized prostate cancer. Magma 2008;21(6):371–7.

13. Heijmink SW, Fütterer JJ, Hambrock T, et al. Prostate cancer: body-array versus endorectal coil MR imaging at 3 T--comparison of image quality, localization, and staging performance. Radiology 2007;244(1):184–95.

14. Zakian KL, Sircar K, Hricak H, et al. Correlation of proton MR spectroscopic imaging with gleason score based on step-section pathologic analysis after radical prostatectomy. Radiology 2005;234(3):804–14.

15. Farrell C, Noyes SL, Joslin J, et al. Prostate multiparametric magnetic resonance imaging program implementation and impact: initial clinical experience in a community based health system. Urol Pract 2018;5:165–71.

16. Schiavina R, Bianchi L, Mineo Bianchi F, et al. Preoperative staging with 11C-choline PET/CT is adequately accurate in patients with very high-risk prostate cancer. Clin Genitourin Cancer 2018;16(4):305–12.e1.

17. Van Damme J, Tombal B, Collette L, et al. Comparison of 68Ga-prostate specific membrane antigen (PSMA) Positron emission Tomography computed Tomography (PET-CT) and whole-body magnetic resonance imaging (WB-MRI) with diffusion sequences (DWI) in the staging of advanced prostate cancer. Cancers 2021;13(21):5286.

18. Evangelista L, Bertoldo F, Boccardo F, et al. Diagnostic imaging to detect and evaluate response to therapy in bone metastases from prostate cancer: current modalities and new horizons. Eur J Nucl Med Mol Imaging 2016;43(8):1546–62.

19. Gonzalez-Montoro A, Ullah MN, Levin CS. Advances in detector instrumentation for PET. J Nucl Med 2022;63(8):1138–44.

20. Majewski S, Proffitt J. Dedicated mobile high-resolution prostate PET imager with an insertable transrectal probe. US Patent 2010;7(858):944.

21. Weinberg I. Dedicated apparatus and method for Positron emission Tomography of the prostate. US Patent 2006;134:102.

22. Huh SS, Clinthorne NH, Rogers WL. Investigation of an internal PET probe for prostate imaging. Nucl Instrum Meth A 2007;579:339–43.

23. Gonzalez AJ, Sanchez F, Benlloch JM. Organ-dedicated molecular imaging systems. IEEE Trans Rad Plasma Med Scie 2018;2:388–403.

24. Huber JS, Choong WS, Moses WW. Initial results of a Positron tomograph for prostate imaging. IEEE Trans Nucl Scie 2005;53:2653–9.

25. Cañizares G, Gonzalez-Montoro A, Freire M, et al. Pilot performance of a dedicated prostate PET suitable for diagnosis and biopsy guidance. EJNMMI Physics 2020;7:1–17.

26. Turkington TG, Smith MF, Hawk TC, et al. PET prostate imaging with small planar detectors. IEEE Symposium Conference Record Nuclear Science 2004;2806–9.

27. Delfino EP, Majewski S, Raylman RR, et al. Towards 1mm PET resolution using DOI modules based on dual-sided SiPM readout. IEEE Nuclear Science Symposuim & Medical Imaging Conference 2010;3442–9.

28. Majewski S, Stolin A, Martone P, et al. Dedicated mobile PET prostate imager. J Nucl Med 2011;52:1945.

29. Park SJ, Rogers WL, Huh S, et al. Performance evaluation of a very high-resolution small animal PET imager using silicon scatter detectors. Phys Med Biol 2007;52(10):2807–26.

30. Miyaoka RS, Li X, Hunter WCJ, et al. Design of a time-of-flight PET imaging probe. IEEE Nuclear Science Symposium Conference Record 2011;3661–4.

31. Miyaoka RS, Hunter WCJ, Pierce LA, et al. Optimization of a hybrid PET (HyPET) detector for prostate cancer imaging. IEEE Nuclear Science Symposium and Medical Imaging Conference (NSS/MIC) 2021;1–4.

32. Garibaldi F, Capuani S, Colilli S. TOPEM: a PET-TOF endorectal probe, compatible with MRI for diagnosis and follow up of prostate cancer. Nucl Instrum Meth A 2013;702:13–5.

33. Garibaldi F, Beging S, Canese R, et al. A novel TOF-PET MRI detector for diagnosis and follow up of the prostate cancer. Eur Phys J Plus 2017;132:396.

34. Huber JS, Moses WW, Pouliot J, et al. Dual-modality PET/ultrasound imaging of the prostate. IEEE Nuclear Science Symposium Conference Record 2005; 2187–90.

35. Meyer TC, Endo-TOFPET-US. A multimodal ultrasonic probe featuring time of flight PET in diagnostic and therapeutic endoscopy. Nucl Instrum Meth A 2013;718:121–5.

36. Vandenberghe S, Moskal P, Karp JS. State of the art In total body PET. EJNMMI Physics 2020,7(1).35.

37. Reddin JS, Scheuermann JS, Bharkhada D, et al. Performance evaluation of the SiPM-based Siemens Biograph vision PET/CT system. IEEE Nuclear Science Symposium and Medical Imaging Conference Proceedings (NSS/MIC) 2018;1–5.

38. van Sluis J, de Jong J, Schaar J, et al. Performance characteristics of the digital Biograph vision PET/CT system. J Nucl Med 2019;60(7):1031–6.

39. Surti S. Update on time-of-flight PET imaging. J Nucl Med 2015;56(1):98–105.

40. Gonzalez-Montoro A, Pourashraf S, Cates J, et al. Cherenkov radiation–based coincidence time resolution measurements in BGO scintillators. Front Physics 2022;10:1–12.

41. Konstantinou G, Lecoq P, Benlloch JM, et al. Meta-scintillators for ultrafast gamma detectors: a review of current state and future perspectives. IEEE Trans Rad Plasma Med Scie 2022;6:5–15.

42. Muehlematter UJ, Nagel HW, Becker A, et al. Impact of time-of-flight PET on quantification accuracy and lesion detection in simultaneous 18F-choline PET/MRI for prostate cancer. EJNMMI Res 2018;8(1):41.

43. Burger I, Muehlematter UJ, Nagel H, et al. Impact of time-of-flight PET on lesion detection rate in 18F-Choline PET/MR for prostate cancer. J Nucl Med 2017;58:1081.

44. Badawi RD, Shi H, Hu P, et al. First human imaging studies with the EXPLORER total-body PET scanner. J Nucl Med 2019;60:299–303.

45. Azghadi S, Abdelhafez Y, Parikh M, et al. Detectability rates and impact on management from high-sensitivity total-body 18F-fluciclovine PET/CT scans in patients with prostate cancer biochemical recurrence. Int J Radiat Oncol Biol Phys 2021;111: e264–5.

46. Katal S, Fibschutz I S, Saboury B, et al. Advantages and applications of total-body PET scanning. Diagnostics 2022;12(2):426.

47. Liberini V, Laudicella R, Balma M, et al. Radiomics and artificial intelligence in prostate cancer: new tools for molecular hybrid imaging and theragnostics. Eur Radiol Exp 2022;15:27.

48. Fukushima M, Hattori Y, Yoshizawa T, et al. Combination of non-viral connexin 43 gene therapy and docetaxel inhibits the growth of human prostate cancer in mice. Int J Oncol 2007;30(1):225–31.

49. Osborne JR, Akhtar NH, Vallabhajosula S, et al. Prostate-specific membrane antigen-based imaging. Urol Oncol: Seminars and Original Investigations 2012;31:144–54.

50. Tagawa ST, Beltran H, Vallabhajosula S, et al. Anti-prostate-specific membrane antigen-based radioimmunotherapy for prostate cancer. Cancer 2010;116: 1075–83.

51. Bander NH, Milowsky MI, Nanus DM, et al. Phase I trial of 177lutetium-labeled J591, a monoclonal antibody to prostate-specific membrane antigen, in patients with androgen-independent prostate cancer. J Clin Oncol 2005;23:4591–601.

Innovations in Small-Animal PET Instrumentation

Adrienne L. Lehnert, PhD*, Robert S. Miyaoka, PhD

KEYWORDS

- Preclinical PET • Functional imaging • PET/MR • PET/CT • Spatial resolution

KEY POINTS

- Recent developments in gene editing, immuno-PET, and high-resolution in vivo imaging have only increased the importance of small-animal, or preclinical, PET imaging.
- Drivers of preclinical PET innovation include new combinations of imaging technologies, such as PET/MR imaging, which require changes to PET hardware.
- As preclinical scanner capability continues to approach the relative spatial resolution of human systems, the importance of preclinical PET will only increase.

PET TECHNOLOGY

There is always a balance to be struck when designing PET systems; overall performance depends on spatial resolution, detection sensitivity, and timing performance, all of which are constrained by cost. In the case of preclinical imaging, it is especially important to have excellent spatial resolution, as the critical structures in mice and other small animals are much smaller than in humans. The extent of this issue can be briefly illustrated by the fact that in order to have a sampling density equivalent to 3 mm spatial resolution in humans, the preclinical scanner would need to have a spatial resolution of approximately 0.5 mm for a rat and 0.2 mm for a mouse.[1] The authors explore innovations in PET system performance by examining those in the arenas of PET detector material and geometry, photosensors, and data acquisition methods.

PET Detectors

One of the main drivers of PET spatial resolution comes from the detectors themselves. These detectors, almost always composed of inorganic scintillator crystals, convert the 511-keV photons to visible or near-visible light, which is then read by a photosensor. This is traditionally done using arrays of discrete crystals. This has the advantage of relatively simple spatial decoding; the location of the photon interaction in the crystal is simply determined by identifying the crystal of interaction. Perhaps the most intuitive way to improve spatial resolution is by using as a small diameter crystal as feasible.

The very first "micro-PET" system had 2×2 mm^2 cross-sectional crystals and a reported spatial resolution of 2.0 mm full width at half maximum (FWHM).[2] A few years later the micro-PET II system was announced with 0.955×0.955 mm^2 cross-sectional crystals.[3] Many other systems followed a similar trajectory, leading to multiple prototype systems with crystals with cross sections under 0.5×0.5 mm^2.[4,5] However, constructing arrays of very small crystals significantly degrades sensitivity due to the proportionally large amount of active volume taken up by reflectors or gaps. Furthermore, manufacturing cost is quite high due to most of the scintillator crystal material being lost in the cutting process.

Another important driver of spatial resolution is related to positioning within the discrete crystal

Department of Radiology, University of Washington, 1959 Northeast Pacific Street, UW Box 356043, Seattle, WA, USA
* Corresponding author.
E-mail address: alehnert@uw.edu

PET Clin 19 (2024) 59–67
https://doi.org/10.1016/j.cpet.2023.09.002
1556-8598/24/© 2023 Elsevier Inc. All rights reserved.

elements. Many 511-keV photons will penetrate many millimeters into the scintillator material before undergoing photoelectric absorption. If only a single depth is assumed, the reconstructed image will have blurring related to parallax error, which is especially prevalent in the close geometries of preclinical imaging.[6] Therefore, incorporating depth of interaction (DOI) capabilities is very valuable.

Crystal Geometry and Material

Several groups have explored using monolithic, or semi-monolithic, crystals in preclinical PET systems.[4,7] For the reasons outlined above, these detectors do not have the sensitivity losses of discrete arrays and are easier (and potentially less costly) to manufacture. Using dense photosensor arrays, monolithic crystal designs have the potential to provide very high intrinsic positioning resolution at a much lower cost. Furthermore, it is much easier to decode DOI in monolithic crystals based on the amount of light spread. Their most notable limitation has traditionally been significant positioning bias near the edges of the crystals. There are also disadvantages based on more complex calibration requirements and processing a high number of signal channels. Spatial resolution does degrade with increasing thickness. This can be counteracted using either dual-sided readout or reading only off the entrance side of the crystals.[8–10]

Although most systems based on monolithic crystal geometries use several crystals optically coupled together, an alternative is to make a preclinical imaging system using a single annulus of crystal. This system is read out by arrays of silicon photomultipliers (SiPMs) coupled to outer facets and had an average spatial resolution of less than 1.5 mm in the radial and axial directions.[11] Another group has created a prototype scanner in which the SiPMs are attached to the ends of the monolithic ring instead of the outer facets.[12]

Some designs have used semi-monolithic slat or trapezoidal crystals.[13–16] These detectors arguably have the "the best of both worlds" with the positioning capabilities of discrete arrays in one direction, whereas light spread along the long dimension provides both positioning and DOI information. The slat concept removes the most significant design challenge associated with fully monolithic crystal detectors, positioning along the edges and corners. Edges and corners are eliminated using slats along one dimension. In addition, the investigators have also demonstrated the ability to decode across crystal boundaries when the edges of crystals are optically coupled.[17]

Thus, slat crystal detectors offer outstanding three-dimensional (3D) positioning with virtually no degradation from edge effects. A variant of the slat crystal detector approach, the trapezoidal slat detector, has also been proposed as an alternative geometry to enable very high detector packing fraction for very compact ring diameter PET detector systems.[18] For example, compact PET detector rings for use with preclinical MR imaging systems.

There have also been efforts exploring the detector material in preclinical PET systems. The requirements for PET systems are well understood and include high detection efficiency, and therefore a high attenuation coefficient, good energy resolution for scatter/photopeak discrimination, fast timing for random minimization and potentially time-of-flight information, and rugged materials for ease in machining small crystal elements. Although there are several options in scintillation material such as sodium iodide (NaI:Tl) and bismuth germanate (BGO), many of which are still in use in nuclear medicine, ever since cerium-doped lutetium oxy-orthosilicate (LSO:Ce), and later lutetium-yttrium oxyorthosilicate (LYSO), were developed in the 1990s, they have been the primary choice in clinical and preclinical PET systems.[19,20]

Some groups have also been exploring using the room temperature semiconductor detector cadmium zinc telluride (CZT) as an alternative to inorganic scintillators.[21–24] CZT has benefits in that the detectors can be quite compact, have excellent energy resolution (~3% at 511 keV) and ultrafine spatial resolution. They also have the capability of 3D event positioning, which reduces parallax error. However, they have poor timing resolution and a low atomic number.[25] One way that investigators have compensated to the lower intrinsic detection efficiency is by orienting the detectors in an edge-on geometry that supports very thick detector configurations.[26]

Another technique that has achieved very good spatial resolution (<0.55 mm) in preclinical PET uses mechanical multi-pinhole collimators.[27,28] Although this technique results in very low detection efficiency, utilization of a clustered pinhole pattern can improve efficiency and the high spatial resolution could be useful for detection, quantitation, and localization of very targeted tracers.[4]

Photosensors

All PET systems using scintillators require sensors that convert the visible or near-ultraviolet (NUV) photons into an electrical signal. In small-animal PET, this has been traditionally accomplished using position-sensitive photomultiplier tubes (PSPMTs). However, photomultiplier tubes (PMTs) have a dead area around their outer edges, are quite bulky, and are incompatible with the high magnetic fields found in MR imaging. Although light guides and optical fibers can mitigate some of these disadvantages, solid-state photomultipliers, namely SiPMs, are now the first choice in high-resolution, scintillator-based PET. The process to fabricate SiPMs is inherently less expensive than PMTs. They are much more compact, can operate in magnetic fields, and have very high gain and outstanding response times.[1,4] When first introduced, SiPM technology faced several challenges such as low photon detection efficiency due to limited fill factor and low sensitivity to the blue-green wavelengths produced by scintillators, cross-talk, and high dark count rates.[29,30] However, this technology has been rapidly improving, and most of the newly developed preclinical PET systems use SiPMs. Currently, both analog and digital SiPMs are available.

Depth of Interaction

One of the best ways of preserving the improved spatial resolution is to incorporate DOI information and therefore minimize spatial blurring due to parallax errors. An illustration of parallax error due to DOI is shown in **Fig. 1**. In general, FWHM DOI resolution should be less than 1 mm to support less than 0.5-mm FWHM spatial resolution.[4] As discussed above, monolithic detector designs inherently provide DOI information in their light response. Semiconductor detectors are pixelated in three dimensions and can also easily provide interaction positioning in the detector array. For discrete crystal scintillators, there are three main strategies for DOI determination: (1) phoswich detector, (2) differential light sharing, and (3) dual-sided readout.[31–36] A more extensive discussion of DOI techniques can be found in the earlier chapter of this publication titled "Advances in PET detectors and readout technologies."

The most common method is the phoswich detector in which multiple layers of discrete crystals with different light responses are used to separate the detector into two or more depth bins.[37–42] These layers may have different crystal materials, so that they can be differentiated by the light decay times, or be offset spatially such that light is shared differently depending on the layer of interaction. Although this is a relatively straightforward and economical method to extract DOI information, it requires additional effort in system fabrication and is limited to two-to-four DOI bins.[4,43]

In differential light sharing, the reflectors between crystal elements are constructed such that the amount of light shared with its neighbor depends on interaction depth. This has the benefit of providing a continuous estimate of DOI along the crystal, but significantly increases calibration and fabrication efforts, especially with crystals with cross sections less than 1×1 mm^2.[36] One variation of this concept uses a single crystal that has been partially subdivided using subsurface laser etching in such a way that differential light sharing between segments provides DOI.[14,44–46] Another variation of this concept is to couple a prismatic light guide to the entrance surface of the crystal for controlled and deterministic light sharing.[47] This single-sided-readout system was able to achieve DOI resolutions of 2.5 mm FWHM in their four-to-one crystal-to-pixel coupled detector modules.[47]

The third and best-performing technique for DOI determination in discrete crystals requires placing sensors on two or more sides of the discrete crystal array. This is usually the entrance and rear surfaces. Using this technique, several systems have achieved better than 2 mm FWHM.[2,48–50]

Signal Multiplexing

With the wider adoption of SiPMs versus PSPMTs in PET applications, multiplexing has become an area of significant interest. This is because one of the technical challenges with SiPM-based or other position-sensitive detectors is the large

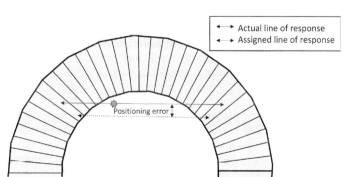

← Actual line of response
←···► Assigned line of response

Positioning error

Fig. 1. Illustration of parallax error in a truncated PET detector ring. Lack of depth of interaction information leads to error in determining the correct line of response.

number of output channels coming from the array. This can easily overload the subsequent data acquisition electronics and limits scalability of the system. Reducing of the number of output channels through strategic combinations of SiPM outputs can significantly ease data processing. However, this must be balanced with issues surrounding increased pulse pile-up and dead time when events must share signal pathways.[7,51,52]

Strategies for signal multiplexing can be based on modulating charge, time, frequency, or polarity. Charge modulation is perhaps the best known of the multiplexing strategies. Here, the input charge collected from SiPM arrays is modulated based on charge division multiplexing networks. An early version of this, Anger logic, was used in PMT arrays. Now, it is more common to see discretized positioning circuits (DPCs) in PET detector systems. A DPC uses a 2D resistive chain to steer toward the four DPC nodes. Hybrid DPCs use a combination of resistors and capacitors and provide better timing performance over conventional DPCs.[51] Another simple form of charge modulation-based multiplexing is row–column sum, which avoids some of the SiPM cross talk of DPMs, but requires more channels. Simple row–column summing can be significantly improved through strategic grouping of channels. Principal component analysis techniques have been demonstrated to reach or even exceed FWHM performance with no multiplexing.[53,54]

Time-modulating multiplexing method operates on a similar philosophy as charge multiplexing methods, except instead of relative ratios of charge, the nodes measure differences in time distance of arrival (TDOA) to decode the primary SiPM element. Different techniques can be used to introduce delays in the signal, although the network designs are relatively simple, highly precise time measurements are required and bulky coaxial cables are not practical.[51] Multiplexing strategies based on frequency or polarity modulation have also been proposed and could reduce channels down by a further 50% to 75% in the case of polarity modulation or even to a single channel with frequency modulation. However, they are currently limited by scalability and count rate performance factors.[51]

PRECLINICAL MULTIMODALITY SCANNER CONFIGURATIONS

One major driver for innovations in preclinical PET technology is the increased interest in multimodality imaging systems. Research PET/CT scanners have been commercially available since the early 2000s, but it took another 10 years or so for PET/MR imaging machines to be commercially available. The advent of solid state photomultipliers had a profound effect on making combined PET/MR systems a reality. Other potentially useful configurations combine PET with optical, single-photon emission computed tomography (SPECT), and integrated radiotherapy.

PET/MR Imaging

As mentioned above, the implementation of SiPM technology in PET systems has been instrumental in the development of PET/MR scanners, both in clinical and preclinical arenas. One challenge in clinical PET/MR lies in the lack of direct measurement of photon attenuation provided by a CT and therefore difficulties in correcting for 511-keV attenuation in the patient. However, this is less of a concern in small-animal imaging, and the benefit MR imaging brings to soft tissue contrast outweighs the lack of PET attenuation correction. Other advancements benefiting the spread of preclinical PET include small footprint, permanent magnet MR imaging systems that do not require cryogenic cooling and reach strengths up to 7 T. These systems are less expensive and easier to maintain than earlier cryogenic scanners and do not require the additional radio frequency (RF) shielding and special ventilation facility modifications. Some systems have integrated PET with MR, whereas others use a PET insert that can be used as stand-alone PET or within the MR scanner. Another manufacturer has a PET detector system that can be coupled to the outside of the MR imaging units ("MR Solutions"). Other vendors use the strategy of cassettes that can be moved between compatible scanners while maintaining animal configuration.

PET/Single-Photon Emission Computed Tomography

The development of preclinical SPECT/CT roughly paralleled that of PET/CT. The mechanical integration of these systems was somewhat similar and even led to the creation of tri-modality PET/SPECT/CT systems.[4,25] These systems were commercially available and were particularly popular in the mid-2000s. Although PET/SPECT/CT combined scanners are still available, it is more common to see dual-modality scanners or systems of multiple small desktop scanners that use standardized cassettes to transfer animals between scanners while keeping the same relative positioning (Molecubes, SOFIE, MR Solutions, and Mediso). These systems benefit from being able to image multiple animals at the same time.

Another strategy is to use the same detector for both PET and SPECT. This allows for simultaneous dual-tracer imaging, opening the door to new clinical and preclinical applications, such as perfusion–metabolism differential imaging of neurodegenerative diseases or two receptor binding studies.[41,55–57] These systems use a cylindrical collimator inserted between the detectors and bed and can achieve submillimeter spatial resolution in both modalities.[57]

PET/Optical

Like in the case of hybrid PET/SPECT imaging, PET/optical fusion imaging is motivated by the desire to measure multiple molecular targets simultaneously. Optical methods using bioluminescent or fluorescent reporter genes, or optical probes, are used extensively in the preclinical arena but are largely not translatable to humans. Combining optical and nuclear medicine radiotracer studies provides the translational platform between preclinical and clinical studies. Some efforts are underway to develop simultaneous PET/optical systems using inserts or mirrors.[4,58,59] Another strategy is to use clear mouse holders that are shaped and sized to hold an animal in an immobilized and geometrically defined position so that it may be imaged in separate scanners.[60] This also allows for easier segmentation because the reproducible animal positioning closely matches that of an atlas.[61]

RESEARCH APPLICATIONS OF PRECLINICAL PET

Motion Correction and Awake Animal Imaging

Motion correction in human studies is generally aimed at correcting for the involuntary movement due to respiratory and cardiac activity. This usually takes the form of signal gating or data-driven corrections. Preclinical systems may use similar techniques to compensate for animal respiration and cardiac activity. However, there is interest in correcting for animal movement during awake, unrestrained imaging, especially in neuroimaging studies.[62–64] This is partially motivated by the desire to do behavioral studies, and partially because of the confounding effect of anesthetics in preclinical PET.[65] Although efforts were made to make a wearable rat PET scanner,[66] most systems now rely on correcting for motion in the awake animal. This can be done with the use of video cameras and visual fiduciary markers,[63] or by attaching point sources to the animal's head.[67,68]

Multiple Animal Imaging

One of the challenges in wider use of preclinical PET is the high relative cost for a single animal

dose and scanner time. Because of the overhead involved in making a dose, it costs about the same to make one mouse dose of approximately 300 µCi as it does for 10 doses. However, because scans can take a significant portion of the 110 minute ^{18}F half-life and doses are limited to very small volumes, it is difficult to get more than three to four imaging sessions out of a single dose order. Therefore, if the imaging bore is large enough, it is useful to image multiple animals at once. Several groups have constructed "hotels" that allow imaging of 2, 4, or potentially more mice at one time.[69–71] Although imaging multiple animals makes better use of available resources, challenges remain in injecting multiple animals, physiologic monitoring, and anesthesia.

PET + Radiation Therapy

One application that is commonly used in the clinic but has not yet made it to the preclinical arena is the integration of PET/CT into radiotherapy. The combination of functional and anatomic images with the therapy machine is vital for tumor delineation to guide the therapy irradiator, as higher tumor doses and improved sparing of healthy tissue provide much better outcome. A couple of small PET/CT systems that can be integrated into existing animal irradiators have been built and are undergoing testing.[8,72] The two irradiators that are commercially available, X-RAD SmART (Precision X-ray, Inc, North Branford, CT) and SAARP (Small Animal Radiotherapy Research Platform from Xstrahl Life Sciences developed at Johns Hopkins University), each have onboard imaging capabilities, but these are 2D or 3D bioluminescent imaging and do not provide the level of functional imaging available with PET.[73] Furthermore, successful integration of PET/CT with radiotherapy could pave the way toward adaptive radiotherapy that accounts for changes during treatment due to tumor growth, regression, or weight loss. The functional information provided by PET would also guide dose boosting to areas with high fluorodeoxyglucose F18 (FDG) uptake or hypoxia.[73]

Another area in which integrated PET/RT would be helpful is in proton therapy range verification via imaging positron emitters resulting from proton-induced nuclear interactions during proton therapy. Such imaging may improve treatment accuracy, allow reduction of radiation margins, and enhance the therapeutic ratio of proton therapy.[74–76]

CLOSING THOUGHTS

Thanks to the enormous potential in novel immuno-PET tracers, it is highly likely that the use of PET in the preclinical arena is only going to increase. This will grow the market for simple-to-use benchtop PET/CT or PET/MR that can be operated by scientists with little imaging background. Other strategies that allow researchers to conveniently image more animals without sacrificing quantitation by lowering per-animal tracer costs will be vital. Innovations that allow for rapid data and image analysis, perhaps using artificial intelligence, will also drive down the cost for preclinical PET. Perhaps the largest impact that imaging researchers can have is to push for ways to reach ~0.2-mm FWHM PET image resolution. This level of spatial resolution, which would require effective motion correction, would enable mouse neuro-PET imaging in new and exciting ways.

CLINICS CARE POINTS

- Understanding relative performance characteristics between preclinical and clinical PET scanners will become more important as the use of co-clinical trials for drug development continues to grow.

DISCLOSURE

The authors have nothing to disclose.

ACKNOWLEDGEMENTS

We want to thank the many funding sources that have supported us over the years including: NIH National Cancer Institute (Grant No. R01 CA136569), NIH National Institute for Biomedical Imaging and Bioengineering (Grant Nos. R01 EB002117, R21/R33 EB0001563, R21 EB013716), Department of Energy (Grant No. DOE DE-FG02-08ER64668), General Electric Medical Systems, Philips Medical Systems, Zecotek Photonics and Altera Corporation.

REFERENCES

1. Adler SS, Seidel J, Choyke PL. Advances in preclinical PET. Semin Nucl Med 2022;52(3):382–402.
2. Cherry SR, Shao Y, Silverman RW, et al. MicroPET: a high resolution PET scanner for imaging small animals. IEEE Trans Nucl Sci 1997;44(3):1161–6.
3. Tai YC, Chatziioannou AF, Yang Y, et al. MicroPET II: design, development and initial performance of an improved microPET scanner for small-animal imaging. Phys Med Biol 2003;48(11):1519–37.
4. Miyaoka RS, Lehnert AL. Small animal PET: a review of what we have done and where we are going. Phys Med Biol 2020;65(24):24TR04.
5. Godinez F, Gong K, Zhou J, et al. Development of an ultra high resolution PET scanner for imaging rodent paws: PawPET. IEEE Transactions on Radiation and Plasma Medical Sciences 2018;2(1):7 16.
6. Levin CS, Zaidi H. Current trends in preclinical PET system design. Pet Clin 2007;2(2):125–60.
7. Gonzalez-Montoro A, Gonzalez AJ, Pourashraf S, et al. Evolution of PET detectors and event positioning algorithms using monolithic scintillation crystals. IEEE Transactions on Radiation and Plasma Medical Sciences 2021;5(3):282–305.
8. Cheng X, Hu K, Yang D, et al. A compact and lightweight small animal PET with uniform high-resolution for onboard PET/CT image-guided preclinical radiation oncology research. Phys Med Biol 2021;66(21):215003.
9. Miyaoka RS, Li X, Lockhart C, et al. Comparison of detector intrinsic spatial resolution characteristics for sensor on the entrance surface and conventional readout designs. IEEE Trans Nucl Sci 2010;57(3):990–7.
10. Maas MC, Schaart DR, Laan DJ, Jan) van der, Lemaître C, Beekman FJ, van Eijk CWE. Monolithic scintillator PET detectors with intrinsic depth-of-interaction correction. Phys Med Biol 2009;54(7):1893.
11. Freire M, Gonzalez-Montoro A, Cañizares G, et al. Experimental validation of a rodent PET scanner prototype based on a single LYSO crystal tube. IEEE Transactions on Radiation and Plasma Medical Sciences 2022;6(6):697–706.
12. Xu J, Xie S, Zhang X, et al. A preclinical PET detector constructed with a monolithic scintillator ring. Phys Med Biol 2019;64(15):155009.
13. Barrio J, Cucarella N, Freire M, et al. Characterization of a PET detector based on semi-monolithic crystals. In: 2021 IEEE nuclear science Symposium and medical imaging conference. NSS/MIC); 2021. p. 1–3. https://doi.org/10.1109/NSS/MIC44867.2021.9875553.
14. Kang HG, Nishikido F, Tashima H, et al. A novel approach for trapezoid geometry small animal DOI PET detector using SSLE technique. J Nucl Med 2019;60(supplement 1):528.
15. Miyaoka RS, Hunter WCJ, Lehnert AL. A better MoUSE Trap detector. IEEE nuclear science symposium and medical imaging conference (NSS/MIC); 2014. p. 1–4. https://doi.org/10.1109/NSSMIC.2014.7430869.
16. Chung YH, Lee SJ, Baek CH, et al. New design of a quasi-monolithic detector module with DOI capability for small animal pet. Nucl Instrum Methods Phys Res Sect A Accel Spectrom Detect Assoc Equip 2008;593(3):588–91.
17. Morrocchi M, Hunter WCJ, Guerra AD, et al. Evaluation of event position reconstruction in monolithic crystals that are optically coupled. Phys Med Biol 2016;61(23):8298–320.

18. Yang Y, James SS, Wu Y, et al. Tapered LSO arrays for small animal PET. Phys Med Biol 2010;56(1):139–53.

19. Melcher CL, Schweitzer JS. Cerium-doped lutetium oxyorthosilicate: a fast, efficient new scintillator. IEEE Trans Nucl Sci 1992;39(4):502–5.

20. Pepin CM, Perrot AL, Berard P, et al. Investigation of the properties of new scintillator LYSO and recent LSO scintillators for phoswich PET detectors. IEEE Nuclear Science Symposium Conference Record 2002;2:655–60.

21. Yu AR, Park SJ, Choi YY, et al. Performance characterization of a new CZT-based preclinical SPECT system: a comparative study of different collimators. J Inst Met 2015;10(09):P09016.

22. Abbaszadeh S, Levin CS. New-generation small animal positron emission tomography system for molecular imaging. J Med Imaging 2017;4(1):011008.

23. Jin Y, Streicher M, Yang H, et al. Experimental evaluation of a 3-D CZT imaging spectrometer for potential use in compton-enhanced PET imaging. IEEE Transactions on Radiation and Plasma Medical Sciences 2023;7(1):18–32.

24. Groll A, Stanford-Hill R, Levin CS. Performance assessment of a high-resolution small animal CZT PET system. IEEE nuclear science symposium and medical imaging conference (NSS/MIC); 2021. p. 1–3. https://doi.org/10.1109/NSS/MIC44867.2021.9875718.

25. Amirrashedi M, Zaidi H, Ay MR. Advances in preclinical PET instrumentation. Pet Clin 2020;15(4):403–26.

26. Peng H, Levin CS. Recent developments in PET instrumentation. Curr Pharm Biotechnol 2010;11(6):555–71.

27. Beekman F, van der Have F. The pinhole: gateway to ultra-high-resolution three-dimensional radionuclide imaging. Eur J Nucl Med Mol Imag 2007;34(2):151–61.

28. Walker MD, Ooorden MC, Dinelle K, et al. Performance assessment of a preclinical PET scanner with pinhole collimation by comparison to a coincidence-based small-animal PET scanner. J Nucl Med 2014;55(8):1368–74.

29. Herbert DJ, Saveliev V, Belcari N, et al. First results of scintillator readout with silicon photomultiplier. IEEE Trans Nucl Sci 2006;53(1):389–94.

30. Herbert DJ, Moehrs S, D'Ascenzo N, et al. The silicon photomultiplier for application to high-resolution positron emission tomography. Nucl Instrum Methods Phys Res Sect A Accel Spectrom Detect Assoc Equip 2007;573(1):84–7.

31. Derenzo SE, Moses WW, Jackson HG, et al. Initial characterization of a position-sensitive photodiode/BGO detector for PET (positron emission tomography). CA (USA): Lawrence Berkeley Lab; 1988. Available at: https://www.osti.gov/biblio/6353824. Accessed April 6, 2023.

32. Moses WW, Virador PRG, Derenzo SE, et al. Design of a high-resolution, high-sensitivity PET camera for human brains and small animals. IEEE Trans Nucl Sci 1997;44(4):1487–91.

33. Shao Y, Cherry SR. A study of depth of interaction measurement using bent optical fibers [in PET scanner]. IEEE Trans Nucl Sci 1999;46(3):618–23.

34. Dokhale P, Stapels C, Christian J, et al. Performance measurements of a SSPM-LYSO-SSPM detector module for small animal positron emission tomography. IEEE nuclear science symposium conference record (NSS/MIC); 2009. p. 2809–12. https://doi.org/10.1109/NSSMIC.2009.5401653.

35. Ito M, Hong SJ, Lee JS. Positron emission tomography (PET) detectors with depth-of- interaction (DOI) capability. Biomed Eng Lett 2011;1(2):70.

36. Ito M, Lee MS, Lee JS. Continuous depth-of-interaction measurement in a single-layer pixelated crystal array using a single-ended readout. Phys Med Biol 2013;58(5):1269.

37. Wong WH. Designing a stratified detection system for PET cameras. IEEE Trans Nucl Sci 1986;33(1):591–6.

38. Yamashita T, Watanabe M, Shimizu K, et al. High resolution block detectors for PET. IEEE Trans Nucl Sci 1990;37(2):589–93.

39. Tsuda T, Murayama H, Kitamura K, et al. A four-Layer depth of interaction detector block for small animal PET. IEEE Trans Nucl Sci 2004;51(5):2537–42.

40. Kang HG, Tashima H, Nishikido F, et al. Initial results of a mouse brain PET insert with a staggered 3-layer DOI detector. Phys Med Biol 2021;66(21):215015.

41. Yao R, Deng X, Beaudoin JF, et al. Initial evaluation of LabPET/SPECT dual modality animal imaging system. IEEE Trans Nucl Sci 2013;60(1):76–81.

42. Pepin CM, Berard P, Perrot AL, et al. Properties of LYSO and recent LSO scintillators for phoswich PET detectors. IEEE Trans Nucl Sci 2004;51(3):789–95.

43. Niu M, Liu Z, Kuang Z, et al. Ultra-high-resolution depth-encoding small animal PET detectors: using GAGG and LYSO crystal arrays. Med Phys 2022;49(5):3006–20.

44. Miyaoka RS, Lewellen TK, Yu H, et al. Design of a depth of interaction (DOI) PET detector module. IEEE Trans Nucl Sci 1998;45(3):1069–73.

45. Hunter WCJ, Miyaoka RS, MacDonald L, et al. Light-sharing interface for dMiCE detectors using sub-surface laser engraving. IEEE Trans Nucl Sci 2015;62(1):27–35.

46. Uchida H, Sakai T, Yamauchi H, et al. A novel single-ended readout depth-of-interaction PET detector fabricated using sub-surface laser engraving. Phys Med Biol 2016;61(18):6635–50.

47. Cao X, Labella A, Zeng X, et al. Depth of interaction and coincidence time resolution characterization of ultrahigh resolution time-of-flight prism-PET modules. IEEE Transactions on Radiation and Plasma Medical Sciences 2022;6(5):529–36.

48. Yang Y, Bec J, Zhou J, et al. A prototype high-resolution small-animal PET scanner dedicated to mouse brain imaging. J Nucl Med 2016;57(7): 1130–5.

49. Kuang Z, Wang X, Fu X, et al. Dual-ended readout small animal PET detector by using 0.5 mm pixelated LYSO crystal arrays and SiPMs. Nucl Instrum Methods Phys Res Sect A Accel Spectrom Detect Assoc Equip 2019;917:1–8.

50. Lee MS, Cates JW, Gonzalez-Montoro A, et al. High-resolution time-of-flight PET detector with 100 ps coincidence time resolution using a side-coupled phoswich configuration. Phys Med Biol 2021; 66(12):125007.

51. Park H, Yi M, Lee JS. Silicon photomultiplier signal readout and multiplexing techniques for positron emission tomography: a review. Biomed Eng Lett 2022;12(3):263–83.

52. LaBella A, Petersen E, Cao X, et al. 36-to-1 multiplexing with prism-PET for high resolution TOF-DOI PET. J Nucl Med 2021;62(supplement 1):38.

53. Pierce LA, Hunter WCJ, Haynor DR, et al. Multiplexing strategies for monolithic crystal PET detector modules. Phys Med Biol 2014;59(18): 5347–60.

54. Pierce LA, Pedemonte S, DeWitt D, et al. Characterization of highly multiplexed monolithic PET/gamma camera detector modules. Phys Med Biol 2018; 63(7):075017.

55. Shao Y, Yao R, Ma T, et al. Initial studies of PET-SPECT dual-tracer imaging. IEEE Nuclear Science Symposium Conference Record 2007;6:4198–204.

56. Bartoli A, Belcari N, Del Guerra A, et al. Simultaneous PET/SPECT imaging with the small animal scanner YAP-(S)PET. IEEE Nuclear Science Symposium Conference Record 2007;5:3408–13.

57. Goorden MC, van der Have F, Kreuger R, et al. VECTor: a preclinical imaging system for simultaneous submillimeter SPECT and PET. J Nucl Med 2013; 54(2):306–12.

58. Li C, Yang Y, Mitchell GS, et al. Simultaneous PET and multispectral 3-dimensional fluorescence optical tomography imaging system. J Nucl Med 2011; 52(8):1268–75.

59. Cherry SR. Multimodality imaging: beyond PET/CT and SPECT/CT. Semin Nucl Med 2009;39(5): 348–53.

60. Klose A, Paragas N. Systems and methods for imaging of an anatomical structure. Published online October 29, 2020. Accessed April 5, 2023. https://patents.google.com/patent/US2020033781 9A1/en.

61. Klose AD, Paragas N. Automated quantification of bioluminescence images. Nat Commun 2018;9(1): 4262.

62. Kyme AZ, Fulton RR. Motion estimation and correction in SPECT, PET and CT. Phys Med Biol 2021; 66(18):18TR02.

63. Kyme AZ, Judenhofer MS, Gong K, et al. Open-field mouse brain PET: design optimisation and detector characterisation. Phys Med Biol 2017;62(15): 6207–25.

64. Enríquez-Mier-y-Terán FE, Brandt O, Kwon SI, et al. Open-Field mouse brain PET: towards a system for simultaneous brain PET and behavioral analysis in small animals. 2021 IEEE nuclear science symposium and medical imaging conference (NSS/MIC); 2021. p. 1–3. https://doi.org/10.1109/NSS/MIC44867.2021. 9875774.

65. Miranda A, Bertoglio D, Stroobants S, et al. Translation of preclinical PET imaging findings: challenges and motion correction to overcome the confounding effect of anesthetics. Front Med 2021;8:753977.

66. Woody C, Kriplani A, O'Connor P, et al. RatCAP: a small, head-mounted PET tomograph for imaging the brain of an awake RAT. Nucl Instrum Methods Phys Res Sect A Accel Spectrom Detect Assoc Equip 2004;527(1):166–70.

67. Miranda A, Glorie D, Bertoglio D, et al. Awake 18F-FDG PET imaging of memantine-induced brain activation and test–retest in freely running mice. J Nucl Med 2019;60(6):844–50.

68. Arias-Valcayo F, Herraiz JL, Galve P, et al. Awake preclinical brain PET imaging based on point sources. 15th International Meeting on Fully Three-Dimensional Image Reconstruction in Radiology and Nuclear Medicine 2019;11072:546–50.

69. Aide N, Visser EP, Lheureux S, et al. The motivations and methodology for high-throughput PET imaging of small animals in cancer research. Eur J Nucl Med Mol Imag 2012;39(9):1497–509.

70. Keller SH, L'Estrade EN, Dall B, et al. Quantification accuracy of a new HRRT high throughput rat hotel using transmission-based attenuation correction: a phantom study. 2016 IEEE nuclear science symposium, medical imaging conference and room-temperature semiconductor detector workshop (NSS/MIC/RTSD); 2016. p. 1–3. https://doi.org/10. 1109/NSSMIC.2016.8069467.

71. Greenwood HE, Nyitrai Z, Mocsai G, et al. High-Throughput PET/CT imaging using a multiple-mouse imaging system. J Nucl Med 2020;61(2): 292–7.

72. Cheng X, Yang D, Saha D, et al. Integrated small animal PET/CT/RT with onboard PET/CT image guidance for preclinical radiation oncology research. Tomography 2023;9(2):567–78.

73. Ghita M, Brown KH, Kelada OJ, et al. Integrating small animal irradiators with functional imaging for

advanced preclinical radiotherapy research. Cancers 2019;11(2):170.

74. Shao Y, Sun X, Lou K, et al. In-beam PET imaging for on-line adaptive proton therapy: an initial phantom study. Phys Med Biol 2014;59(13):3373.

75. Parodi K, Assmann W, Belka C, et al. Towards a novel small animal proton irradiation platform: the SIRMIO project. Acta Oncologica 2019;58(10):1470–5.

76. Zhong Y, Lu W, Chen M, et al. Novel online PET imaging for intrabeam range verification and delivery optimization: a simulation feasibility study. IEEE Transactions on Radiation and Plasma Medical Sciences 2020;4(2):212–7.

High-resolution Imaging Using Virtual-Pinhole PET Concept

Yuan-Chuan Tai, PhD[a,b,c],*

KEYWORDS

- Positron emission tomography • PET • Virtual-pinhole PET • Zoom-in PET imaging
- Organ-specific PET imaging

KEY POINTS

- Virtual-pinhole PET concept leads to novel PET system designs that can optimize the performance (including image resolution, system sensitivity, and imaging field-of-view [FOV]) of organ-specific PET scanners.
- Virtual-pinhole PET insert technology enables high-resolution zoom-in PET imaging capability using clinical whole-body PET/CT scanners.
- Virtual-pinhole PET systems can provide high-resolution PET images for any organ-of-interest without compromising the whole-body imaging FOV of a clinical PET/CT scanner.

INTRODUCTION

PET with ^{18}F-fluorodeoxyglucose (FDG) has proven success in measuring glucose metabolism in heart and brain[1,2] as well as finding metastatic cancer diseases,[3,4] taking advantage of the increased aerobic glycolysis (Warburg effect[5]) in cancer cells. Whole-body FDG-PET/computed tomography (CT)[6,7] is used clinically to scan a patient from the base of the skull to the thighs for cancer staging and restaging, as well as for monitoring response to therapy.[8–10] Driven by this demand, clinical PET/CT scanners are optimized for whole-body imaging using large rings of detectors to accommodate a patient's body. The image resolution of PET is known to be limited by (1) positron range of the radionuclides, (2) the acolinearity of the annihilation gamma rays, and (3) the intrinsic spatial resolution of PET detectors.[11] With a ring diameter of greater than 80 cm, the photon acolinearity effect (ie, the 2 gamma rays from a positron annihilation are not emitted along a straight line) limits the image resolution of a whole-body PET scanner to be no better than ~2 mm full-width-at-half-maximum (FWHM). Constructing a whole-body PET scanner with expensive high-resolution PET detectors does not improve the overall image resolution effectively. This is particularly true when the image quality is often count-limited rather than resolution-limited when using a whole-body imaging protocol. As a result, improvement in whole-body PET scanners has not been focused on detector intrinsic resolution but noise reduction (eg, time-of-flight (TOF) PET[12]), MR/PET capability,[13] and ultra-high sensitivity[14,15] in recent years, despite submillimeter resolution PET detectors being available for preclinical imaging applications.

Virtual-pinhole PET is a system design concept that places PET detectors strategically in an unconventional geometry to optimize the performance of PET for specific imaging tasks.[16] Using this concept, one may place high-resolution PET detectors close to an organ-of-interest to achieve

[a] Department of Radiology, Washington University in St. Louis, St Louis, MO, USA; [b] Department of Biomedical Engineering, Washington University in St. Louis, St Louis, MO, USA; [c] Department of Electrical and System Engineering, Washington University in St. Louis, St Louis, MO, USA
* Washington University School of Medicine, Campus Box 8225, 510 South Kingshighway Boulevard, St Louis, MO 63110.
E-mail address: taiy@wustl.edu

PET Clin 19 (2024) 69–82
https://doi.org/10.1016/j.cpet.2023.08.002
1556-8598/24/© 2023 Elsevier Inc. All rights reserved.

the highest image resolution and/or system sensitivity; and then place additional detectors away from the target region to overcome the geometric constraints imposed by human anatomy. An asymmetric geometry permits one to mix detectors of different characteristics (eg, different dimensions, intrinsic spatial resolution, efficiency, and so forth) in a system to optimize the desired performance while minimize the overall system cost. Importantly, virtual-pinhole PET concept has led to the invention of PET devices that can enable "zoom-in PET imaging"[17,18] using an existing PET scanner.[19] This approach offers the benefits of organ-specific PET scanners (ie, higher image resolution and system sensitivity) through the use of an optional accessory device that can be attached to a clinical whole-body PET/CT scanner on demand[20]—a potentially more cost-effective solution to support innovative applications that require higher spatial resolution than

detector in array 1 and all the detectors in array 2 in **Fig. 1**B, these LORs form a fan beam geometry that allows the radioactivity distribution in an object to be "projected" onto the surface of array #2 with a magnification. The magnification factor depends on the ratio of d_1 and d_2 (ie, the distances from the object to the 2 detector arrays). To achieve a higher magnification, one would place the detector array 1 close to an object at the expense of a reduced imaging field-of-view (FOV). This is similar to a pinhole camera with which one can trade imaging FOV for resolution by adjusting the object-to-pinhole distance "b" in **Fig. 1**A.

The image resolution of a virtual-pinhole PET system (R_{sys}) is still limited by the 3 fundamental physical factors previously described and can be expressed as follows:[16]

$$R_{sys} \approx \sqrt{R_{src}^2 + R_{180^\circ}^2 + R_{set}^2}$$

$$\approx \sqrt{R_{src}^2 + \left[0.0088 \bullet \frac{d_1 \bullet d_2}{(d_1 + d_2)}\right]^2 + \left[\frac{d_2 \bullet w_1 + d_1 \bullet w_2 + |d_2 \bullet w_1 - d_1 \bullet w_2|}{2 \bullet (d_1 + d_2)}\right]^2} \tag{1}$$

that can be offered by a whole-body PET scanner. This article describes the basic concept of virtual-pinhole PET and uses several novel PET system designs as examples to illustrate its potential applications. The advantages and limitations of virtual-pinhole PET designs relative to the standard whole-body PET scanners and other dedicated organ-specific PET systems will also be discussed.

FUNDAMENTALS OF VIRTUAL-PINHOLE PET

Virtual-pinhole PET concept uses a magnifying geometry that is similar to a pinhole camera to achieve high-resolution PET imaging. **Fig. 1**A illustrates a simplified pinhole camera containing a gamma camera and a pinhole collimator while **Fig. 1**B shows a simplified virtual-pinhole PET system containing 2 detector arrays of different sizes (and intrinsic spatial resolution) that are placed at different distances from the object. A pinhole collimator restricts the direction of gamma rays that can reach the γ-camera surface in order to form a projection image. A PET scanner uses coincidence detection to determine the direction of the annihilation gamma rays without the need of a physical collimator. Consider the coincidence line-of-response (LOR) connecting the single

where, R_{src} is the effective source dimension including the positron range effect, R_{180° is the blurring from photon acolinearity effect, and R_{det} is the detector's intrinsic spatial resolution. The object-to-detector distances (d_1 and d_2) and detector widths (w_1 and w_2) are defined in **Fig. 1**B in the unit of millimeter. When an object is very close to detector array #1 (ie, $d_1 \ll d_2$), the term R_{180° approaches $0.0088 \cdot d_1$ while the term R_{det} approaches w_1. That is, the blurring due to photon acolinearity effect is determined primarily by the shorter of the 2 object-to-detector distances while the image resolution of the system is limited primarily by the intrinsic spatial resolution of the detector array #1 near the object. This is, again, analogous to a pinhole camera whose image resolution is limited by the pinhole size instead of the intrinsic spatial resolution of the camera when $b \ll f$ in **Fig. 1**A. If one considers the high-resolution detector #1 as a "virtual-pinhole," the image resolution of a virtual-pinhole system is bounded by the "virtual-pinhole size," which corresponds to the intrinsic spatial resolution of detector array #1. If the array #1 contains multiple detector elements, the system in **Fig. 1**B is effectively a "virtual multipinhole" PET camera that preserves both the resolution benefits of a magnifying pinhole geometry and the sensitivity benefits of

B

Detector array 2

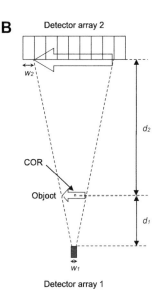

w_2

d_2

COR

Object

d_1

w_1

Detector array 1

A

γ-camera

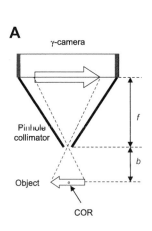

Pinhole collimator

f

b

Object

COR

Fig. 1. (*A*) A simplified pinhole single photon emission computed tomography (SPECT) system consists of a gamma camera and a pinhole collimator that can be rotated around a center-of-rotation. (*B*) A simplified virtual-pinhole PET system consists of a high-resolution detector array (#1) and a low-resolution detector array (#2) that can be rotated around a center-of-rotation. (This research was originally published in JNM. Yuan-Chuan Tai, Heyu Wu, Debashish Pal, Joseph A. O'Sullivan. Journal of Nuclear Medicine Mar 2008, 49 (3) 471-479 © SNMMI.)

PET through coincidence detection (without the need of a physical collimator).

To obtain tomographic images using the virtual-pinhole PET concept, one could rotate a pair of detectors around an object as illustrated in **Fig. 2**A or rotate a high-resolution PET detector inside an existing PET scanner[21] (**Fig. 2**B and C) to collect coincidence events for 360° or 180° sampling. Alternatively, one could insert a full-ring of high-resolution PET detectors inside an existing PET scanner (**Fig. 3**) to enhance its image resolution within a reduced imaging FOV.[19,22]

With a full ring of high-resolution PET detectors placed inside the imaging FOV of an existing PET scanner, coincidence events may be detected by a pair of the insert detectors (namely the insert-insert or II events, represented by blue LOR in **Fig. 4**), or a pair of the native scanner detectors (namely the scanner-scanner or SS events represented by the black LOR), or between an insert detector and a scanner detector (namely the IS events represented by the red LOR), provided that the insert detectors do not stop all 511-keV gamma rays. The II and SS events in **Fig. 4** are essentially from 2 conventional PET scanners with different ring diameters whose image resolution is determined by their corresponding detector intrinsic spatial resolution and ring diameter. The IS events follow the virtual-pinhole PET geometry in **Fig. 1** whose image resolution is described by Eq. (1). To achieve the best image resolution and system sensitivity, one could establish a system matrix that models the detector response of all 3 types of events for joint image reconstruction.

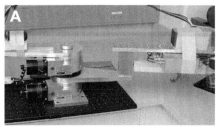
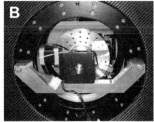
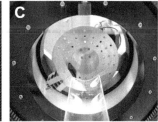

Fig. 2. (*A*) An the experimental setup of a simplified virtual-pinhole PET system consists of a high-resolution detector array on the left and a low-resolution detector array on the right that can be rotated around an object at the center of the rotation stages. This research was originally published in JNM. Yuan-Chuan Tai, Heyu Wu, Debashish Pal, Joseph A. O'Sullivan. Journal of Nuclear Medicine Mar 2008, 49 (3) 471-479. © SNMMI. (*B*) A high-resolution PET detector array mounted to a rotation stage that is attached to the back side of a microPET scanner. This research was originally published in JNM. Heyu Wu, Debashish Pal, Joseph A. O'Sullivan, Yuan-Chuan Tai, A Feasibility Study of a Prototype PET Insert Device to Convert a General-Purpose Animal PET Scanner to Higher Resolution, Journal of Nuclear Medicine Dec 2007, 79-87. © SNMMI. (*C*) Front view of the insert device. The add-on detector is positioned closed to the central axis of the scanner to resemble the virtual-pinhole PET geometry. (*Adapted from* the Journal of Nuclear Medicine with Permission. DOI:10.2967/jnumed.107.043034 and DOI:10.2967/jnumed.107.044149.)

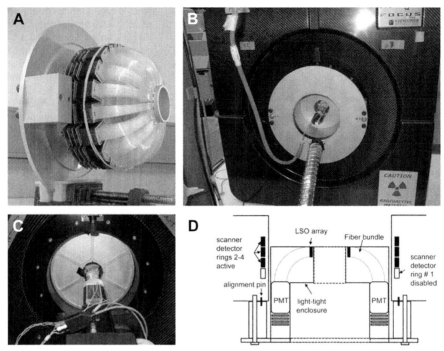

Fig. 3. A virtual-pinhole PET device with a full-ring of high-resolution PET detectors mounted to an existing animal PET scanner: (*A*) the device with its cover removed; (*B*) the device mounted to the back of a microPET F-220 scanner Concorde Microsystems Inc. (Knoxville, TN); (*C*) front view of scanner with the device attached. The animal port opening is reduced to 5.4 cm in diameter; (*D*) position of high-resolution detector ring relative to the detector rings in the native scanner. (This research was originally published in JNM. Heyu Wu et al. Micro Insert: A Prototype Full-Ring PET Device for Improving the Image Resolution of a Small Animal PET Scanner. J Nucl Med. Year;49:1668–1676. © SNMMI.)

Fig. 5 shows images of a micro-Derenzo phantom that was scanned by the prototype system in **Fig. 3** and reconstructed using the II, IS, or SS events individually or jointly. As expected, the II image exhibits the highest spatial resolution but also most noisy. The SS image has the lowest resolution but less noisy. The jointly estimated images (II + IS, or II + IS + SS) achieve better resolution than the native scanner (represented by the SS image) and less noise than using the high-resolution detectors alone (represented by the II image).

This example demonstrates that one can mix detectors of different characteristics to design a PET system using the virtual-pinhole PET concept. The additional flexibility presents new opportunities to innovate in application-specific or organ-specific PET systems with expanded imaging FOV.[23–25] Furthermore, the virtual-pinhole PET insert technology was expanded to enable high-resolution zoom-in imaging capability using existing whole-body PET/CT scanners.[20,26] The following examples illustrate new opportunities in high-resolution organ-specific PET innovations enabled by the virtual-pinhole PET concept.

EXPAND THE FIELD-OF-VIEW OF BREAST PET IMAGER BY THE VIRTUAL-PINHOLE PET CONCEPT

Most positron emission mammography (PEM) systems place high-resolution PET detectors closely around one or both breasts, arranged in either planar or ring geometry, to maximize the overall system sensitivity. The imaging FOV of such PEM systems is limited to the breast tissues only because the placement of PET detectors is constrained by human anatomy. Lesions inside the chest wall are undetectable. Breast tissues near the chest are viewable by limited number of detectors resulting in suboptimal image quality due to low system sensitivity in this region. Lesions in the axilla may be detected if additional detectors are placed at an (or multiple) oblique angle(s) to extend the imaging FOV. Using conventional geometry, PEM systems offer high-resolution images and high system sensitivity with some limitations in imaging FOV.

Using the virtual-pinhole PET concept, Tai and colleagues evaluated the feasibility of a dedicated

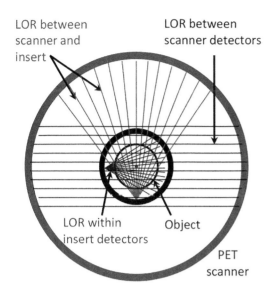

LOR between scanner and insert

LOR between scanner detectors

LOR within insert detectors

Object

PET scanner

Fig. 4. Three types of coincidence events (II, IS, and SS) may be detected when a set of high-resolution detectors are inserted inside the imaging FOV of a PET scanner.

breast PET imager with an imaging FOV extended beyond the chest wall of a patient. **Fig. 6** illustrates an asymmetric geometry of a PEM system constructed using 2 types of detectors: the small half-ring #1 enclosing a breast is made of high-resolution PET detectors to maximize the image resolution, whereas the large half-ring #2 is made of lower resolution PET detectors to limit the total cost. This system can also register 3 types of coincidence events (II, IS, and SS, represented by red, blue, and green lines in **Fig. 6**A) from radioactivity in the FOV. The central circular FOV encompasses a breast and tissues near and inside the chest wall.

Five point sources within the circular FOV were simulated. Sinogram of the SS, IS, and II types of coincidence events is shown in **Fig. 6**B–D, respectively. None of the individual sinograms provides complete sampling for tomographic image reconstruction. However, the combined sinogram (**Fig. 6**E) shows complete sampling for tissues in the lower half of the circular FOV. For tissues inside the chest wall, the sampling is near complete and can be reconstructed with less artifact, especial if the detectors support TOF PET operation.

Built on this study, Samanta and colleagues proposed a novel "Total Breast PET system,"[25] which offers an imaging FOV encompassing both breasts and the entire torso (**Fig. 7**). The scanner comprises of 2 types of detectors: (1) high-resolution TOF PET detectors capable of resolving the depth-of-interaction (DOI) of gamma rays are used in the anterior panel and stadium ring to achieve the best image resolution and (2) cost-effective TOF PET detectors that have medium resolution and high efficiency (commonly used in clinical PET scanners) are used in the posterior panel to provide large solid-angle coverage of the torso. Coincidence events detected within and between the anterior panel and the stadium ring provide high-resolution PET images of the breasts, similar to that achievable by conventional PEM systems. Coincidence events between these high-resolution detectors and the posterior panel form the virtual pinhole PET geometry, enabling high-resolution PET images in regions near the chest wall and the axilla. Importantly, standard-resolution PET images are also available for the rest of the torso when all coincidence events are used for image reconstruction.

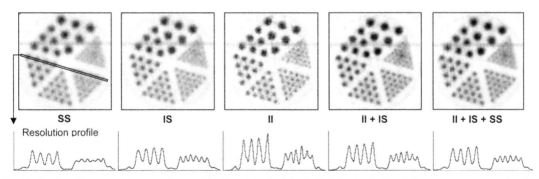

SS IS II II + IS II + IS + SS

Resolution profile

Fig. 5. A micro-Derenzo phantom imaged by the virtual-pinhole PET device in **Fig. 3**. Images were reconstructed using SS, IS, or II coincidence events separately, or jointly. Diameters of the fillable rods in the phantom are 0.8, 1.0, 1.25, 1.5, 2.0, and 2.5 mm, respectively. Profiles through 1-mm and 1.5-mm diameter rods are extracted from each image and shown below. The native scanner resolution (SS images) is improved when coincidence events measured by insert (II or IS) are included for image reconstruction. Jointly reconstructed images are less noisy than the high-resolution insert device alone (II image). (This research was originally published in JNM. Heyu Wu et al. Micro Insert: A Prototype Full-Ring PET Device for Improving the Image Resolution of a Small Animal PET Scanner. J Nucl Med. Year;49:1668–1676. © SNMMI.)

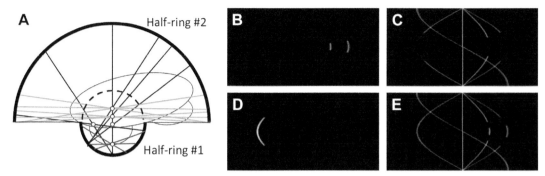

Fig. 6. (*A*) A dedicated PEM system with asymmetric geometry. Five point sources are located at (0, 0), (−10, 0), (0, 6), (0, 10), and (0, −10) (in the unit of centimeter) relative to the origin at the scanner center. Coincidence events detected by lower resolution detectors in the upper half-ring (SS events), between the 2 half-rings (IS events) and by the high-resolution detectors in the lower half ring (II events), are sorted to form the SS, IS, and II sinograms in (*B*), (*C*), and (*D*), respectively. (*E*) A combined sinogram of all events. (*Adapted from* IEEE Transactions on Nuclear Sciences with Permission. DOI: 10.1109/TNS.2006.869853.)

A Monte Carlo simulation study was carried out to compare the performance of the total-breast PET system against a state-of-the-art clinical PET/CT scanner (Siemens Biograph Vision) for the detection of small lesions in the breasts, near axilla, and within the chest wall. **Fig. 8**A i shows the location of 20 lesions inside a simplified torso phantom and 2 breasts. The ratio of the radioactivity concentration between the lesions and the body background ranges from 4:1 to 6:1, whereas the lesion size ranges from 4 to 6 mm in diameter. **Fig. 8**A ii and iii show the map of coincidence events detected by the Biograph Vision scanner and the total-breast PET scanner, respectively. The sensitivity of the total-breast PET scanner is significantly higher than a clinical scanner in the breast regions to provide high-statistics and high-resolution images of the breasts. **Fig. 8**B, C shows substantially higher contrast recovery by the total-breast PET system for all lesions in the breast, regardless of the lesion size or lesion-to-background activity ratio. For the axilla and

regions inside the chest wall, the total-breast PET system is comparable to or better than a clinical whole-body PET/CT scanner.

Using the virtual-pinhole PET concept, the total-breast PET system provides high-resolution breast images achievable only by dedicated PEM systems and a large imaging FOV achievable only by whole-body PET scanners. Although the use of standard PET detectors in the posterior panel reduces the cost of the total-breast PET system when compared with a system made entirely by the high-resolution DOI detectors, additional cost-saving is possible if the posterior panel is substituted by PET detectors in an existing PET/CT scanner. This is illustrated by the next 2 examples using the virtual-pinhole PET insert technology.

VIRTUAL-PINHOLE PET INSERT FOR HEAD-AND-NECK IMAGING

A prototype virtual-pinhole PET insert device was developed and integrated with a Siemens

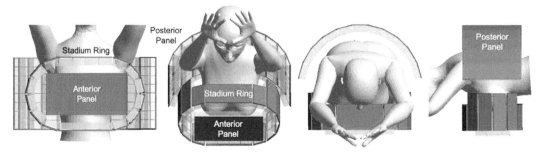

Fig. 7. A total-breast PET imager constructed using 3 groups of detectors: anterior panel and "stadium"-shaped ring contain TOF and DOI capable high-resolution PET detectors while the posterior panel consists of TOF detectors similar to those used in clinical PET/CT systems. (*Adapted from* Physics in Medicine and Biology with Permission. DOI:10.1088/1361-6560/abfb16.)

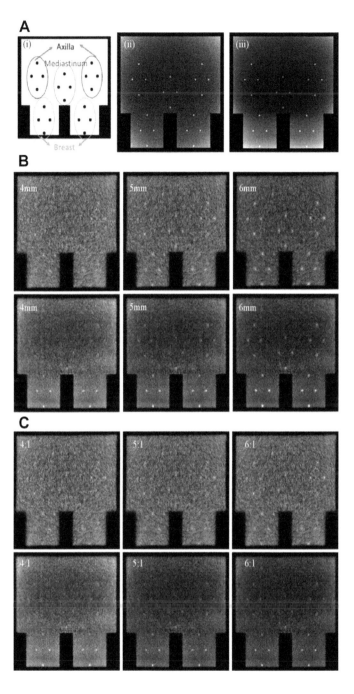

Fig. 8. (*A*) Distribution of coincidence events detected by (ii) Biograph Vision PET scanner and (iii) the total-breast PET imager for lesion diameter 4 mm, 4:1 lesion-to-background ratio (L:B). Lesion placement map shown at left (i). (*B*) Iteratively reconstructed central-slice images of the torso phantom containing lesions of indicated sizes in each image, along with fixed L:B of 4:1 imaged by (top row) whole-body scanner and (bottom row) dedicated total-breast PET scanner. (*C*) Lesions with various indicated L:B along with a fixed lesion diameter of 4 mm imaged by (top row) whole-body scanner and (bottom row) dedicated total-breast PET scanner. (*Adapted from* Physics in Medicine and Biology with Permission. DOI:10.1088/1361-6560/abfb16.)

Biograph 40 PET/CT scanner Siemens Healthineers (Knoxville, TN) to improve its image resolution within a smaller FOV (**Fig. 9**). The Biograph 40 scanner contains 192 PET detectors arranged in 4 rings of 855 mm in diameter. Each detector consists of an array of lutetium oxyorthosilicate (LSO) crystals with 13-by-13 elements each measuring $4 \times 4 \times 20$ mm^3. The virtual-pinhole PET insert device contains 28 detector modules (**Fig. 10A**) that are mounted inside a custom gantry (**Fig. 10B**) to form 2 half-rings of 249 mm in diameter, concentric with the PET/CT scanner's detector rings. Each insert detector module contains an LSO array with 13-by-13 crystals each measuring $2 \times 2 \times 5$ mm^3. Thus, the intrinsic spatial resolution of the insert detectors is approximately 50% of that of the native detectors in both the transverse and the axial directions.

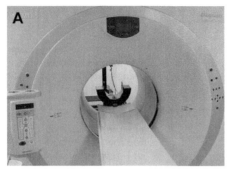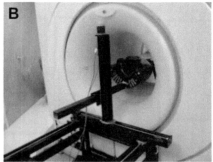

Fig. 9. A Siemens Biograph 40 PET/CT scanner with a prototype virtual-pinhole PET insert attached: (*A*) front view and (*B*) rear view. The virtual-pinhole PET insert gantry is supported by a 3D translation stage that positions the insert detectors concentrically with the scanner's detector rings.

Coincidence detection between the virtual-pinhole PET insert and the native PET scanner was established by reassigning the readout electronics and data channels of 28 (out of the 192) native PET detector modules to the insert detectors. From the list mode data, coincidence events are sorted into 3 groups: II, IS, and SS. A maximum-likelihood expectation-maximization (MLEM) algorithm was developed for joint image reconstruction using all 3 types of events.[26–28] System normalization and correction techniques that account for the attenuation and scattering of gamma rays by the insert detectors are incorporated for image reconstruction.[28–30]

Fig. 11 shows the transverse and sagittal images of Ge-68 line sources (1.8 mm inner diameter and 3.3 mm outer diameter) that are scanned using the Biograph 40 PET/CT scanner (top) or the same scanner with the virtual-pinhole PET insert attached (bottom). Line profiles across the lower 3 line sources in the sagittal view are extracted and shown on the right. The FWHM of the 3 line sources ranges from 4.7 to 5.8 mm in the native scanner image and 3.0 to 3.5 mm in the virtual-

pinhole PET insert image, respectively. Compensating for the size of the Ge-68 source, the image resolution of the Biograph 40 scanner is estimated to range from 4.3 to 5.5 mm FWHM. This is consistent with the performance reported in the literature.[31] In comparison, the image resolution of the virtual-pinhole PET insert device is estimated to range from 2.4 to 3.0 mm FWHM. This represents a reduction of the image resolution by more than 40% in all 3 directions within a reduced imaging FOV.

Fig. 12 shows a patient with cancer in the oropharynx imaged by the Biograph 40 PET/CT scanner (top) followed by the virtual-pinhole PET insert device (bottom). It should be noted that the Biograph 40 PET/CT has a 220-mm axial FOV while the virtual-pinhole PET insert system has a 164-mm axial FOV due to 28 disabled native detectors. Furthermore, the high-resolution insert detectors only cover approximately 6 cm of the central region of the axial FOV. Therefore, the virtual-pinhole PET images were acquired using 2 bed positions. Despite the reduced system sensitivity, the virtual-pinhole PET insert system exhibits

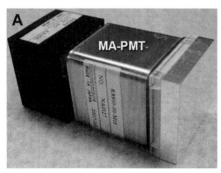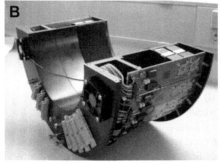

Fig. 10. (*A*) The virtual-pinhole PET insert detector module contains an LSO array (13 × 13 elements) optically coupled to a multi-anode photomultiplier (MA-PMT) via a custom light guide. (*B*) Twenty-eight detector modules are arranged in a custom gantry to form 2 half-rings of 249 mm in diameter. (*With permission from* Hamamatsu Photonics K.K.)

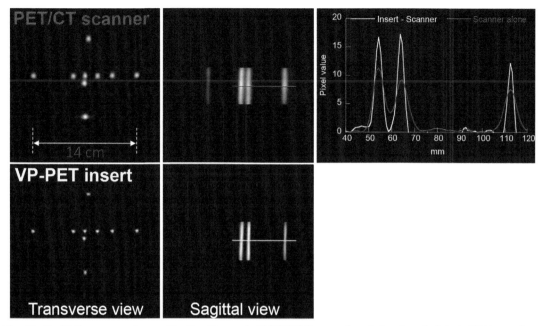

Fig. 11. Ge-68 line sources imaged by the Biograph 40 PET/CT (top row) and the virtual-pinhole PET insert (bottom row). Profiles through 3 line sources show significant improvement in image resolution (>40% reduction in FWHM) when the virtual-pinhole PET insert device is attached to the PET/CT scanner.

better image resolution and higher tumor-to-background contrast than the native PET scanner in this preliminary result.

VIRTUAL-PINHOLE PET INSERT FOR HIGH-RESOLUTION BREAST IMAGING

Leveraging the virtual-pinhole PET insert prototype in **Fig. 9**, Mathews and colleagues developed techniques to locally enhance PET image resolution without compromising the imaging FOV of a whole-body PET scanner.[32] First, Monte Carlo simulation was used to study a simplified torso phantom (with a breast) imaged using a half-ring insert in a body scanner shown in **Fig. 13**A. Six groups of spherical tumors were placed in or near the breast, as shown in **Fig. 13**B. These tumors were 2, 3, 4, 6, 8, and 12 mm in diameter ($\varnothing$), respectively. The tumor-

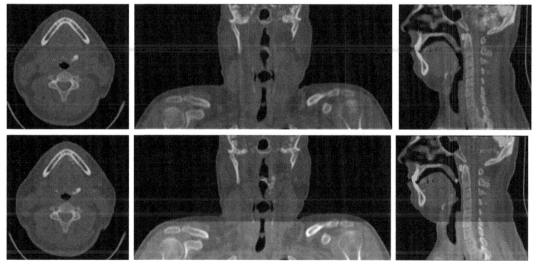

Fig. 12. (Top) PET/CT images of a patient with head and neck cancer scanned by a Biograph 40 scanner. (Bottom) The same patient imaged by the prototype virtual-pinhole PET insert device.

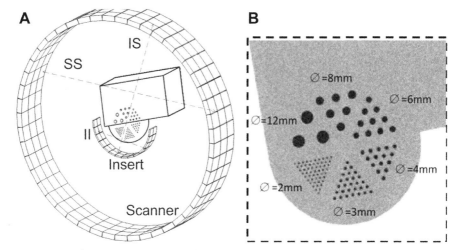

Fig. 13. (*A*) Geometry of the Monte Carlo simulation study using the prototype virtual-pinhole PET insert for breast imaging. (*B*) Magnified view of the breast region showing 6 groups of spherical tumors (2, 3, 4, 6, 8, and 12 mm in diameter, respectively). T/B ratio was 3, 6, 9, or 12. Simulated acquisition time was 2.26 or 6.78 minutes. (*Adapted from* Physics in Medicine and Biology with Permission. doi:10.1088/0031-9155/58/18/6407.)

to-background (T/B) ratio was set to 3, 6, 9, or 12. The simulated acquisition time was 2.26 minutes for a low-statistics scan or 6.78 minutes for a high-statistics scan. The activity concentration in the body background was 5.3 kBq/mL (143 nCi/mL), based on the assumption of 10 mCi of FDG uniformly distributed in a 70 kg patient. The PET/CT scanner simulated was a Siemens Biograph-40 with or without the above virtual-pinhole PET insert prototype attached.

Images were reconstructed using all 3 types of events by an MLEM algorithm that models the

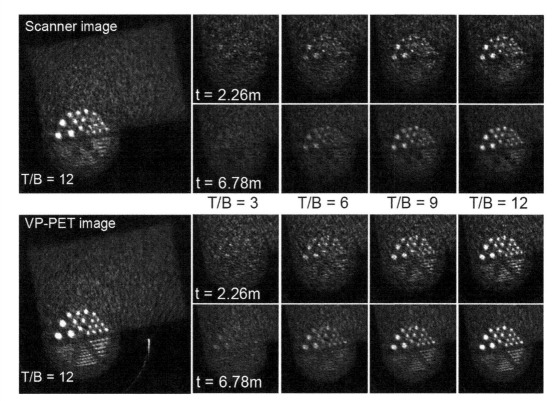

Fig. 14. (Top) Images from the native PET scanner. (Bottom) Images from the virtual-pinhole PET insert system. (*Adapted from* Physics in Medicine and Biology with Permission. doi:10.1088/0031-9155/58/18/6407.)

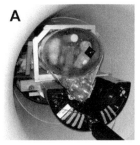 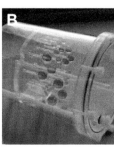 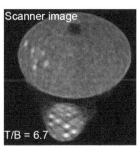 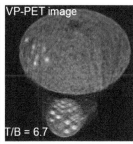

Fig. 15. (*A*) A torso phantom with a breast compartment was imaged using the virtual-pinhole PET insert proto-type in a Biograph 40 PET/CT scanner. (*B*) The breast compartment contains 6 clusters of spherical lesions with their size ranging from 3.3 to 11.4 mm in diameter. The virtual-pinhole PET images (right) exhibit higher resolution in the breast and axilla region than the native scanner images (left). (*Adapted from* Physics in Medicine and Biology with Permission. doi:10.1088/0031-9155/58/18/6407.)

virtual-pinhole PET insert geometry and accounts for additional attenuation and scattering by the insert detectors.[26,28] Results in **Fig. 14** show that (1) a virtual-pinhole PET insert can improve the image resolution of a target region (eg, a breast and its surrounding tissues in this case) while preserving the whole body imaging capability of a PET scanner and (2) with T/B = 3, it will be difficult to detect a tumor 12 mm Ø or smaller using a clinical PET/CT scanner even with a 6.78-minute acquisition time. In contrast, the virtual-pinhole PET insert can detect the 12 mm Ø tumors if the counting statistics are high (eg, in a 6.78-minute scan); (3) with T/B = 6, the scanner can detect 8 mm Ø tumors in a 6.78-minute scan, whereas the virtual-pinhole PET can detect the same size of tumors in a 2.26-minute scan. Alternatively, the virtual-pinhole PET can detect smaller (6 mm Ø) tumors in a 6.78-minute scan; (4) with T/B = 9 or 12, the virtual-pinhole PET can detect 4 mm Ø tumors more reliably than the scanner regardless how long the subject is scanned; and (5) under all conditions, a scanner with the virtual-pinhole PET insert attached outperforms the scanner itself.

Following the Monte Carlo study, a torso phantom with a breast attachment and spherical tumors was imaged experimentally using the prototype virtual-pinhole PET insert, as shown in

Fig. 15A. The breast compartment contains 6 clusters of spherical lesions with their size ranging from 3.3 to 11.4 mm in diameter, arranged in the Derenzo-like pattern. Additional spherical lesions with their size ranging from 3.6 to 11.4 mm in diameter are inserted in the axilla region of the torso phantom. The T/B ratio was 6:1. The results are consistent with the Monte Carlo study above, except that the 4.3-mm diameter lesions in the breast compartment are not as clearly resolved by the prototype device as those by the Monte Carlo simulated system. This is likely due to alignment error between the 2 physical systems and machining error of the insert detector modules and gantry that resulted in an imperfect system model.[32] The lesions in the axilla also seem sharper in the virtual-pinhole PET images demonstrating the resolution benefits of the insert device extended beyond the breast region into the chest and axilla.

VIRTUAL-PINHOLE PET INSERT TECHNOLOGY TO ZOOM-IN ANY ORGAN-OF-INTEREST

Although the proof-of-concept virtual-pinhole PET insert device showed promise in high-resolution head-and-neck and breast imaging applications, its implementation has several limitations: (1) the

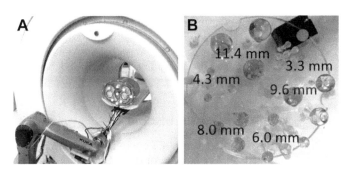

Fig. 16. (*A*) The second-generation virtual-pinhole PET insert system comprises of compact high-resolution PET detectors in a flat-panel enclosure that can be positioned anywhere around a patient's body by a robotic arm. (*B*) Six clusters of spherical lesions are embedded in a torso phantom and filled with radioactivity with blue dye. The activity concentration has a 6:1 T/B ratio. (*Adapted from* Medical Physics with Permission. doi:10.1002/mp.13724.)

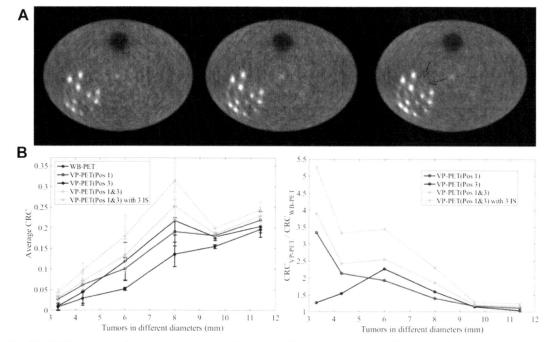

Fig. 17. (*A*) From left to right are native scanner image, and images reconstructed using combined datasets when the insert device was placed below and to the left of the phantom to mimic a dual-panel virtual-pinhole PET insert device, and a dual-panel DOI-capable virtual-pinhole PET insert device that can triple the number of IS events; (*B*) the CRC curves for different configurations (Left) and the CRC ratios with and without the virtual-pinhole PET insert (Right). (*Adapted from* Medical Physics with Permission. doi:10.1002/mp.13724.).

insert detectors use existing readout electronics in the scanner, which requires 28 of the native detectors to be disabled and results in reduced overall system sensitivity; (2) the detectors were constructed using MA-PMT resulting in a bulky gantry and unnecessary attenuation and scattering of signal; (3) the half-ring geometry of the insert offers little flexibility to image other organs of interest; and (4) the location of the insert detectors is fixed in the scanner requiring a patient to be positioned to fit the insert, thus very user-unfriendly. In the second generation virtual-pinhole PET insert system,[20] these limitations were resolved by the following: (1) include additional readout electronics to support the external insert detectors; (2) improve the compactness of the insert detectors using silicon photomultiplier; (3) adapt a flat panel geometry to increase the flexibility in conforming to patient anatomy; and (4) use a robotic arm to support and position the flat-panel insert detectors around a patient's body for any organ of interest. **Fig. 16**A shows the system used to image a torso phantom. Spherical lesions in **Fig. 16**B are filled with radioactivity with a concentration of 6:1 T/B ratio and inserted into the torso phantom. Coincidence events were acquired when the flat-panel insert detectors were initially positioned below the torso phantom, and subsequently

move to the lower left, left, and to the right of the phantom by the robotic arm. Images were reconstructed using a list-mode MLEM reconstruction algorithm implemented using graphic processing unit (GPU).[33] **Fig. 17**A shows the native scanner image (left), virtual-pinhole PET insert image using data acquired from position 1 and 3 to mimic a dual-panel system (middle), and virtual-pinhole PET insert image assuming a dual-panel system made of DOI detectors with higher sensitivity (right). **Fig. 17**B shows the contrast recovery coefficient (CRC) of the lesions is improved when the virtual-pinhole PET insert is incorporated to work in conjunction with a clinical PET/CT scanner. The improvement is most significant if the insert device has dual-panel and high-sensitivity DOI detectors. The relative improvement of the CRC against the native scanner is most prominent for lesions of small diameters, suggesting that the virtual-pinhole PET insert technology may improve the detectability and diagnostic accuracy for small and hard-to-detect lesions.

SUMMARY AND DISCUSSIONS

The virtual-pinhole PET concept offers new opportunities in the design of dedicated organ-specific

PET systems or accessary insert devices to enable zoom-in imaging using existing PET/CT scanners. For the former, a system can be designed from scratch with vast flexibility in the choice of detector technologies considering the tradeoffs between the overall performance and cost. For the latter, communication and coincidence detection between the native scanner and the virtual-pinhole PET insert device may dictate the choice of detector technologies and readout electronics when designing a virtual-pinhole PET insert device that is compatible with existing PET/CT scanners. For newer generation of clinical PET/CT scanners, the option to receive additional (digital or analog) signals from external detectors will accelerate the adaptation of the virtual-pinhole PET insert technology. Furthermore, an industry-wide standard that defines the communication protocol and data format of singles events detected by a system may enable a third party company to design the next-generation virtual-pinhole PET insert devices that can work with PET/CT scanners from multiple vendors — a model similar to that has been used by the vendors of MR surface coils.

With a group of high-density detectors in the imaging FOV of a PET/CT scanner, many standard data correction techniques need to be revalidated or (sometimes) redeveloped. These may include but not limited to attenuation correction, scatter correction, normalization, dead-time model, and so forth. Alignment of the virtual-pinhole PET insert detectors, both spatially and timing-wise, to the native scanner also poses a challenge. This is particularly true if the insert detectors have ultra-high spatial resolution, requiring the spatial alignment of the 2 systems to be less than 1 mm accuracy. Many of these technical challenges can be alleviated if the device integration is incorporated into the design of a clinical PET/CT scanner to support additional accessory detectors. With proper design, the virtual-pinhole PET insert technology can offer a cost-effective solution to bring ultra-high resolution PET imaging capability to human imaging research and clinical applications in the near future.

CLINICS CARE POINTS

- Organ-specific high-resolution PET scanners may offer new opportunities and innovative applications of new radiopharmaceuticals.
- Conventional organ-specific PET scanners offer limited imaging FOV for very specific applications, limiting their wide acceptance clinically as they are incompatible with the standard-of-care FDG whole-body PET/CT imaging.
- The virtual-pinhole PET insert technology can enable zoom-in PET imaging using clinical whole-body PET/CT scanners, thus deliver the best of both worlds: the high-resolution PET images that are available only through organ-specific PET imagers and the large whole-body imaging capability from clinical PET/CT scanners.

DISCLOSURE

The authors have nothing to disclose.

FUNDING

The technologies described in this article were supported by the National Institute of Health through grant awards CA110011, CA136554 and CA233912. The author would also like to acknowledge the grant support from the Susan G. Komen Breast Cancer Foundation (BCTR0601279) and the Siteman Cancer Center (Breast Cancer Developmental Research Awards).

REFERENCES

1. Gallagher BM, Ansari A, Atkins H, et al. Radiopharmaceuticals XXVII. 18F-labeled 2-deoxy-2-fluoro-d-glucose as a radiopharmaceutical for measuring regional myocardial glucose metabolism in vivo: tissue distribution and imaging studies in animals. J Nucl Med 1977;18(10):990–6.

2. Kuhl DE, Phelps ME, Hoffman EJ, et al. Initial clinical experience with 18F-2-fluoro-2-deoxy-d-glucose for determination of local cerebral glucose utilization by emission computed tomography. Acta Neurol Scand Suppl 1977;64:192–3.

3. Gallagher BM, Fowler JS, Gutterson NI, et al. Metabolic trapping as a principle of oradiopharmaceutical design: some factors resposible for the biodistribution of [18F] 2-deoxy-2-fluoro-D-glucose. J Nucl Med 1978;19(10):1154–61.

4. Som P, Atkins HL, Bandoypadhyay D, et al. A fluorinated glucose analog, 2-fluoro-2-deoxy-D-glucose (F-18): nontoxic tracer for rapid tumor detection. J Nucl Med 1980;21(7):670–5.

5. Warburg O, Wind F, Negelein E. The metabolism of tumors in the body. J Gen Physiol 1927;8:519–30.

6. Dahlbom M, Hoffman EJ, Hoh CK, et al. Whole-body positron emission tomography: Part I. Methods and performance characteristics. J Nucl Med 1992; 33(6):1191–9.

7. Beyer T, Townsend DW, Brun T, et al. A combined PET/CT scanner for clinical oncology. J Nucl Med 2000;41(8):1369–79.

8. Glaspy JA, Hawkins R, Hoh CK, et al. Use of positron emission tomography in oncology. Oncology 1993;7(7):41–55.

9. Nieweg OE, Kim EE, Wong WH, et al. Positron emission tomography with fluorine-18-deoxyglucose in the detection and staging of breast cancer. Cancer 1993;71(12):3920–5.

10. Rege SD, Hoh CK, Glaspy JA, et al. Imaging of pulmonary mass lesions with whole-body positron emission tomography and fluorodeoxyglucose. Cancer 1993;72(1):82–90.

11. Cherry SR, Sorenson JA, Phelps ME. Physics in nuclear medicine. 3rd edition. Philadelphia: SAUNDERS; 2003.

12. Surti S. Update on time-of-flight PET imaging. J Nucl Med 2015;56(1):98–105 [published Online First: Epub Date]|.

13. Wehrl HF, Sauter AW, Judenhofer MS, et al. Combined PET/MR imaging - technology and applications. Technol Cancer Res Treat 2010;9(1):5–20.

14. Berg E, Roncali E, Kapusta M, et al. A combined time-of-flight and depth-of-interaction detector for total-body positron emission tomography. Med Phys 2016;43(2):939 [published Online First: Epub Date]|.

15. Badawi RD, Shi H, Hu P, et al. First human imaging studies with the EXPLORER total-body PET scanner. J Nucl Med 2019;60(3):299–303 [published Online First: Epub Date]|.

16. Tai YC, Wu H, Pal D, et al. Virtual-pinhole PET. J Nucl Med 2008;49(3):471–9.

17. Zhou J, Qi J. Theoretical analysis and simulation study of a high-resolution zoom-in PET system. Phys Med Biol 2009;54(17):5193–208 [published Online First: Epub Date]|.

18. Zhou J, Qi J. Adaptive imaging for lesion detection using a zoom-in PET system. IEEE Trans. Med. Imaging 2011;30(1):119–30 [published Online First: Epub Date]|.

19. Wu H, Pal D, Song TY, et al. Micro Insert: a prototype full-ring PET Device for improving the image resolution of an animal PET scanner. J Nucl Med 2008; 49(10):1668–76.

20. Jiang JY, Li K, Wang Q, et al. A second-generation virtual-pinhole PET device for enhancing contrast recovery and improving lesion detectability of a whole-body PET/CT scanner. Med Phys 2019;46(9): 4165–76 [published Online First: Epub Date]|.

21. Wu H, Pal D, O'Sullivan JA, et al. A feasibility study of a prototype PET insert device to convert a general purpose animal PET scanner to higher resolution. J Nucl Med 2008;49(1):79–87.

22. Janecek M, Wu H, Tai YC. A simulation study for the design of a prototype insert for whole-body PET scanners. IEEE Trans Nucl Sci 2006;53(3):1143–9.

23. Tai YC, Wu HY, Janecek M. Initial study of an asymmetric PET system dedicated to breast cancer imaging. IEEE Trans Nucl Sci 2006;53(1):121–6.

24. Wang Q, Mathews AJ, Li K, et al. A dedicated high-resolution PET imager for plant sciences. Phys Med Biol 2014;59(19):5613–29 [published Online First: Epub Date]|.

25. Samanta S, Jiang J, Hamdi M, et al. Performance comparison of a dedicated total breast PET system with a clinical whole-body PET system: a simulation study. Phys Med Biol 2021;66(11). https://doi.org/ 10.1088/1361-6560/abfb16 [published Online First: Epub Date]|.

26. Mathews AJ, Li K, Komarov S, et al. A generalized reconstruction framework for unconventional PET systems. Med Phys 2015;42(8):4591–609.

27. Pal D, O'Sullivan JA, Wu HY, et al. 2D linear and iterative reconstruction algorithms for a PET-insert scanner. Phys Med Biol 2007;52(14):4293–310.

28. Keesing DB, Mathews A, Komarov S, et al. Image reconstruction and system modeling techniques for virtual-pinhole PET insert systems. Phys Med Biol 2012;57(9):2517–38 [published Online First: Epub Date]|.

29. Komarov SA, Heyu W, Keesing DB, et al. Compton scattering in clinical PET/CT with high resolution half ring PET insert device. IEEE Trans Nucl Sci 2010;57(3):1045–51.

30. Bai B, Li Q, Holdsworth CH, et al. Model-based normalization for iterative 3D PET image reconstruction. Phys Med Biol 2002;47(15):2773–84.

31. Brambilla M, Secco C, Dominietto M, et al. Performance characteristics obtained for a new 3-dimensional lutetium oxyorthosilicate-based whole-body PET/CT scanner with the National Electrical Manufacturers Association NU 2-2001 standard. J Nucl Med 2005;46(12):2083–91.

32. Mathews AJ, Komarov S, Wu H, et al. Improving PET imaging for breast cancer using virtual pinhole PET half-ring insert. Phys Med Biol 2013;58(18): 6407–27 [published Online First: Epub Date]|.

33. Jiang JY, Li K, Komarov S, et al. Feasibility study of a point-of-care positron emission tomography system with interactive imaging capability. Med Phys 2019; 46(4):1798–813.

Whole Gamma Imaging
Challenges and Opportunities

Taiga Yamaya, PhD*, Hideaki Tashima, PhD, Sodai Takyu, PhD, Miwako Takahashi, MD, PhD

KEYWORDS

• PET • Compton camera • WGI • Antibody • Multiple myeloma • Positronium

KEY POINTS

- Compton imaging has been recognized as a possible nuclear medicine imaging method following the establishment of SPECT and PET but its clinical use has not been realized yet.
- Whole gamma imaging (WGI), a combination of PET and Compton imaging, could be the first practical method to bring out the potential of Compton imaging in nuclear medicine.
- With the use of such positron emitters as ^{89}Zr and ^{44}Sc, WGI may enable highly sensitive imaging of antibody drugs for early tumor detection and quantitative hypoxia imaging for effective tumor treatment.
- Some concepts have been demonstrated preliminarily in physics experiments and small animal imaging tests with a developed WGI prototype.

INTRODUCTION

"Scatter is the enemy"—this quotation ascribed to Edward J. Hoffman is true in PET for patient scattering but perhaps not for detector scattering.[1–3] Compton scattering in detectors has a potential to provide angular information of an incoming gamma ray based on the Klein-Nishina formula when a deposited energy value at the Compton scattering point is measured accurately.[4] The activity source position can be localized on the surface of a cone by measuring the event which causes Compton scattering using a scatterer detector and photoelectric absorption in an absorber detector (Fig. 1). This is referred to as Compton imaging, and medical applications of Compton cameras are an important topic.[5] Compton cameras have been developed by many groups, and one of them was recently applied clinically.[6] However, current Compton camera technologies suffer from limited image quality, which is generally much lower than that of PET images due to several limits such as the energy resolution, the sensitivity and the detector coverage (ie, the number of projection angles).

One realization of the combined Compton-PET system has been a multicylinder detector geometry, where the inner detector ring works as a scatterer and the outer detector ring works as an absorber for Compton imaging.[7] PET measurement is also possible by taking the outer-outer coincidence as well as the inner-inner coincidence and the inner-outer coincidence. This concept is known as whole gamma imaging (WGI). Zirconium-89 (^{89}Zr), which emits 909-keV gamma rays about 4 times more frequently than it emits positrons, is a good radionuclide for WGI. As Compton imaging is not influenced by the positron range, Compton imaging may have a chance to outperform PET imaging in terms of spatial resolution. The first WGI prototype successfully showed a 909-keV Compton image of a ^{89}Zr-injected mouse, which was almost equivalent to the PET image obtained from the same ^{89}Zr distribution.[8] Although there is scope for technological improvement in Compton imaging, combined Compton and PET imaging has a merit of enhanced sensitivity even if spatial resolution of the Compton imaging is similar to that of PET. Although data correction methods for Compton imaging (eg, attenuation correction and scatter correction) are

Institute for Quantum Medical Science, National Institutes for Quantum Science and Technology, 4-9-1 Anagawa, Inage-ku, Chiba 263-8555, Japan
* Corresponding author.
E-mail address: yamaya.taiga@qst.go.jp

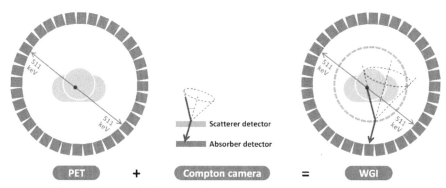

Fig. 1. A conceptual sketch of WGI, which is a novel combination of PET and Compton imaging.

yet to be developed for quantitative imaging, combined Compton and PET imaging is expected to extend systems for clinical use once they have been achieved.

Another potential use of WGI is triple-gamma imaging or β^+-γ coincidence imaging. Scandium-44 (^{44}Sc), which emits a positron (ie, a pair of 511 keV photons) and a 1157-keV γ-ray almost at the same time, is a good example of such a source.[7] The source position can, in principle, be localized at the intersection points between a line-of-response (LOR) and the surface of the Compton cone. This novel direct-imaging method may realize in-situ real-time tracking of tiny activity sources such as a single cell in a regenerative treatment, although further improvement is required in such detector performance parameters as energy resolution, timing resolution, and efficiency to realize the concept.

^{44}Sc-WGI may facilitate realization of positronium (Ps) lifetime imaging, which is a new concept in nuclear medicine.[9] The Ps, a hydrogen-like atom consisting of a positron and an electron, is efficiently formed in the patient body during PET examinations, and its decay rate into 511-keV gamma rays is significantly influenced by the chemical environment, especially the dissolved oxygen concentration due to the unpaired electrons.[10] However, in conventional PET, only radioactivity distribution is used for diagnosis, and nobody has focused on the potential of the Ps lifetime as a biomarker.

PROTOTYPING AND ZIRCONIUM-89 IMAGING

The WGI prototype was developed for a proof-of-concept dedicated to small animal imaging (**Fig. 2**).[8] A whole-body depth-of-interaction (DOI) PET having 4-layer DOI detectors was used as the outer absorber ring. A total of 160 detectors were arranged in 4 subrings, each consisting of 40 detectors. The 4-layer DOI

detectors were equipped with an array of $2.8 \times 2.8 \times 7.5$ mm^3 scintillation crystals (Ce-doped gadolinium oxyorthosilicate codoped with Zr,[11] GSOZ) arranged in a $16 \times 16 \times 4$ configuration, using a layer-by-layer reflector arrangement for three-dimensional (3D) position identification via the Anger-type calculation.[12] Each array of scintillation crystals was coupled to a two-dimensional (2D) multichannel photomultiplier tube. The inner scatterer ring consisted of high-light output scintillation crystals (cerium-doped gadolinium–aluminum–gallium garnet,[13] GAGG) and multipixel photon counters (MPPCs). GAGG crystals $0.9 \times 0.9 \times 6.0$ mm^3 in size were arranged in a 2D array of 24×24. Each crystal array was coupled to an 8×8-array of MPPCs each having a pixel size of 3.0×3.0 mm^2 to form a scatterer detector. A total of 20 scatterer detectors were arranged in 2 subrings, each consisting of 10 detectors.

The WGI prototype not only served as a proof-of-concept but also marked the world's first successful implementation of a full-ring Compton imaging system. For a demonstration of Compton imaging capability, a mouse administered with ^{89}Zr oxalate was measured by the WGI prototype (see **Fig. 2**C). ^{89}Zr emits both positrons and single gamma rays of 909 keV, and therefore, a direct comparison of PET and Compton imaging was possible from the same data. The measurement under an anesthetized condition was performed 22 hours after the 9.8-MBq ^{89}Zr oxalate injection. Because artifact-less 3D Compton imaging requires the entire axial field of view to be covered by the scatterer ring and the axial coverage of the scatterer ring was insufficient for the entire mouse body, the measurement was performed at 2 axial bed positions shifted by 37 mm with a small overlap. The measurement time was 1 hour at each bed position.

The data acquisition (DAQ) system recorded all single events, and data processing, including

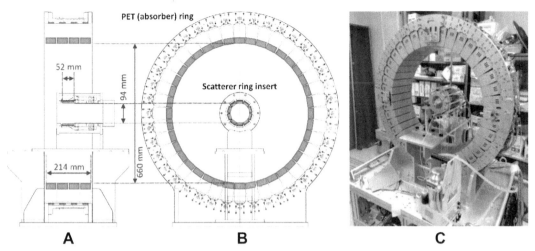

Fig. 2. Design sketches of the WGI prototype side view (*A*) and front view (*B*). Photo showing WGI measurement of a mouse (*C*). Figures A and B were reprinted from the literature[8] under the Creative Commons Attribution 4.0 license.

software coincidence detection, was performed after the measurement. Based on the energy resolution against 511-keV gamma rays, the energy window for PET events was set to 350 to 650 keV for the scatterer with 17% energy resolution and 400 to 600 keV for the absorber with 14% energy resolution.[7] It should be noted that the energy resolution of the scatterer was worse than expected from the scintillator light output due to a mismatch of pulse integration time in the DAQ and light decay time. The energy window for 909-keV Compton events was set to 50 to 350 keV for the scatterer and 550 to 850 keV for the absorber. Another energy window of 800 to 1000 keV was applied for the total energy. The coincidence time window was set to 50 nanoseconds, which is relatively wide because no precise timing correction was applied.

Image reconstruction was performed by the 3D list-mode ordered subset expectation maximization method implemented for WGI Compton imaging.[8] Detector response function (DRF) modeling, normalization (sensitivity correction), and random correction were incorporated. A DRF model was implemented incorporating the angular blurring effect for high-quality image reconstruction. A hollow cylindrical phantom with 5.3 MBq ^{89}Zr solution was measured for 24 hours for normalization. The list-mode data extracted by the software coincidence were used to calculate sensitivity distribution directly in the image domain. The random correction was performed with a delayed coincidence technique with a coincidence window shift of 256 nanoseconds. The same algorithm was applied for PET image reconstruction using the Gaussian model in the LOR DRF modeling.

Fig. 3 compares PET and Compton images. Because the axial length of the absorber (PET) ring was sufficiently long to cover the entire mouse body, the whole mouse body image was obtained with a single bed position. The Compton image was generated by combining 2 images with an axial shift of 37 mm, where position-dependent weight was applied for averaging. It should be noted that although outside the scatter ring, there was a sensitivity for Compton imaging, there were distortions in the reconstructed images due to insufficiency of the data completeness condition for 3D Compton imaging. The result showed that the Compton image quality inside the scatterer ring was approaching PET image quality.

The 909-keV gamma ray emission rate is 4 times more than the positron emission rate. In typical PET measurements, 909-keV gamma rays are a source of noise. Meanwhile, WGI can use 909-keV gamma rays by the Compton Imaging technique. One of the main concepts of WGI is to enhance sensitivity by combining PET and Compton events originating from the same distribution. A hybrid image reconstruction method was developed to realize the WGI concept.[14] The method applied a weighted sum for images individually updated using PET events and Compton events to obtain a hybrid-updated image. To demonstrate the effectiveness of the hybrid method, a low-dose or short-time scan situation was simulated with measured data. **Fig. 4** shows results of a hybrid reconstruction for a 1-minute frame extracted from the 1-hour ^{89}Zr mouse measurement placing the upper body half inside the scatterer ring. Because of the reduced numbers of counts, both PET and Compton images were very noisy compared with the 1-hour

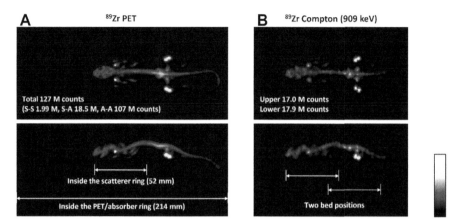

Fig. 3. PET (*A*) and Compton (*B*) images each reconstructed from the same mouse WGI data measured with ^{89}Zr-oxalate injection. The top row shows the maximum intensity projection (MIP) images from the top, and the bottom row shows those from the side. The whole mouse body Compton image was generated by combining 2 images at 2-bed positions. The numbers in the top row images are the measured coincidence event counts. (S-S, scatterer-scatterer; S-A, scatterer-absorber; A-A, absorber-absorber; Upper, the upper body half was inside the scatterer ring; and Lower, the lower body half was inside the scatterer ring.)

measurement results in **Fig. 3** A for the PET images, and **Fig. 3** B for the Compton images. The WGI combining PET and Compton events for image reconstruction showed reduced noise, demonstrating the effectiveness of the hybrid reconstruction method.

RECONSTRUCTION-LESS SCANDIUM-44 IMAGING

Some radioisotopes emit one or more gamma rays at almost the same time as the positron decay. Such radioisotopes are sometimes called triple-gamma nuclides. Taking the coincidence between

a PET event and a Compton event for such triple-gamma nuclides measured by WGI, the emission source position can be identified at the intersection point of the LOR and the Compton cone. Although there are cases where 2 intersection points are inside the field of view, the source position of each coincidence event can be localized at almost a single point without reconstruction. Therefore, reconstruction-less imaging is possible by β^+-γ coincidence with WGI. ^{44}Sc is one of the candidate radionuclides for β^+-γ coincidence imaging. Other candidates are summarized in the literature.[15] To be used in nuclear medicine applications, radionuclides must have a reasonable

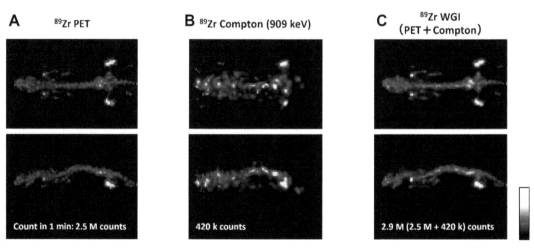

Fig. 4. Demonstration of hybrid image reconstruction combining PET and Compton events as WGI using all detectable events for imaging. (*A*) PET images. (*B*) Compton images. (*C*) WGI images. One-minute data were extracted for the single bed position where the upper body half of the ^{89}Zr-injected mouse was positioned inside the scatter ring. The top row shows MIP images from the top. The bottom row shows MIP images from the side.

half-life (ie, not too short as to prevent easy handling and not too long as to be unsafe).

The source position of a β^+-γ coincidence event consisting of a PET event and a Compton event is calculated using the notations in **Fig 5**. The Compton cone for the Compton event is determined by the scattering angle θ and the line connecting detection positions at the scatterer (**s**) and the absorber (**a**). Let the energy of the original gamma ray energy be E_γ and detection energy at the scatterer be E_s, the scattering angle is determined by the Klein-Nishina equation as

$$\theta = arccos\left(\left(\frac{1}{E_\gamma} - \frac{1}{E_\gamma - E_s}\right)m_e c^2 + 1\right), \quad (1)$$

where m_e is the electron mass and c is the speed of light. Let **c** and **c′** be the detection points of the PET event, **d** be the directional vector from **c** toward **c′**, **n** be the directional vector from **a** toward **s**, and t be the distance between **c** and the intersection point **p** of the LOR and the Compton cone. Then, **p** is determined by solving the following system of equations:

$$\begin{cases} \mathbf{p} = \mathbf{c} + t\mathbf{d} \\ \dfrac{(\mathbf{p} - \mathbf{s}) \bullet \mathbf{n}}{|\mathbf{p} - \mathbf{s}|} = \cos\theta \end{cases} \quad (2)$$

Because the energy information acquired in actual systems contains uncertainty depending on the energy resolution, the calculated scatter angle also contains uncertainty. Considering such uncertainty when drawing the point on the image domain would improve the resulting image quality. Let the variation of the detection energy follow the Gaussian distribution with a standard deviation σ_E. Let the solution of equation (2) be t_0, then, the uncertainty can be modeled using an asymmetric Gaussian function with standard deviations $\sigma^+ = |t^+ - t_0|$ and $\sigma^- = |t^- - t_0|$, where t^+ and t^- are solutions of equation (2) substituting $\theta = \theta^+$ and $\theta = \theta^-$, where θ^+ and θ^- are calculated for varied scatterer detection energy $E_s^+ = E_s + \sigma_E$ and $E_s^- = E_s - \sigma_E$ in equation (1). The asymmetric Gaussian distribution on the LOR is as follows:

$$h(t) = \begin{cases} \dfrac{2}{\sqrt{2\pi}(\sigma^+ + \sigma^-)}\exp\left(-\dfrac{(t - t_0)^2}{2(\sigma^+)^2}\right) & t < t_0 \\[4mm] \dfrac{2}{\sqrt{2\pi}(\sigma^+ + \sigma^-)}\exp\left(-\dfrac{(t - t_0)^2}{2(\sigma^-)^2}\right) & t \geq t_0 \end{cases}$$

$$(3)$$

The LOR also has uncertainty due to the detector element size and other physical limitations of PET spatial resolution. The LOR uncertainty can also be incorporated by modeling the blurring effect into the DRF for PET events. The resulting DRF model for β^+-γ coincidence events is the multiplication of the DRFs for PET and Compton events.

A 166-kBq ^{44}Sc point-like source was measured at offsets from the center to 80 mm with 20 mm steps by the WGI prototype with a scatterer ring had a diameter of 200 mm having 2 subrings of 20 detectors.[7] The measurement time was 120 minutes for each offset. The gamma ray energy of ^{44}Sc is 1157 keV. β^+-γ coincidence events consisting of 4 single events each, including one PET event and one Compton event, were extracted. PET events were extracted only for the absorber-absorber combination with the energy window of 400 to 600 keV. For Compton event extraction, the energy window was 110 to 450 keV for the scatterer, greater than 600 keV for the absorber, and 1000 to 1350 keV for the

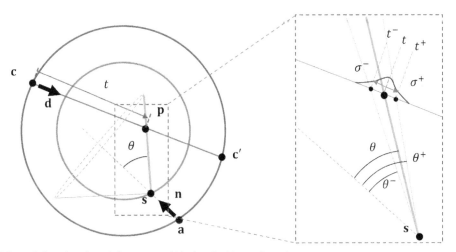

Fig. 5. DRF modeling for the triple gamma (β^+-γ) coincidence imaging.

total energy. The coincidence time window was 20 nanoseconds.

Fig. 6 demonstrates the β^+-γ coincidence imaging of ^{44}Sc compared with a simple LOR backprojection without Compton cone information. The images were generated by summing all the β^+-γ coincidence events for the offsets 0, 20, 40, 60, and 80 mm. The β^+-γ coincidence image showed that background radioactivity could be suppressed without time-consuming image reconstruction, whereas the simple LOR backprojection image showed a strong background. Although the sensitivity of the β^+-γ coincidence is low because it is a multiplication of PET and Compton sensitivities, reconstruction-less imaging has the potential for realizing a real-time imaging application.

POSITRONIUM LIFETIME IMAGING

Ps is an exotic atom that is sometimes formed by a positron binding with an electron before positron-electron annihilation. There are 2 types of Ps: para-positronium (p-Ps) with antiparallel spins and ortho-positronium (o-Ps) with parallel spins. Their production ratio is 1:3. In a vacuum, p-Ps annihilates into 2 photons with the mean lifetime of 125 picoseconds, whereas o-Ps annihilates into 3 photons with the mean lifetime of 142 nanoseconds. The p-Ps lifetime is too short and p-Ps often self-annihilates before interacting with other electrons in a substance. However, the o-Ps lifetime is shortened to 1 to 10 nanoseconds reflecting the surrounding electron density in a substance, and o-Ps finally undergoes 2-photon annihilation (**Fig. 7**). Ps occurs in vivo with a probability of about 30% in PET examinations but its presence is ignored in conventional PET imaging.

Currently, the phenomenon of shortening the Ps lifetime (mainly o-Ps lifetime) in a substance is widely used as an analytical technique to examine the free volume of polymers and the pore size of metals in the field of materials science. The o-Ps lifetime can be measured by using multiple radiation detectors and a radioactive source that emits a prompt gamma ray immediately after β^+ decay such as ^{22}Na. As the half-life of ^{22}Na ($\sim$2.6 years) is too long for its use in nuclear medicine, ^{44}Sc, whose half-life is about 4 hours, is an alternative for future clinical use. A histogram of the detection time difference is obtained by treating the detection of a 1157 keV (for ^{44}Sc) prompt gamma ray as a start and the detection of a 511 keV pair annihilation photon as a stop. The time at which the number of counts in the histogram decreases to 1/e, that is, the o-Ps mean lifetime, is calculated by fitting.

Although measured changes of the Ps lifetime have been used to investigate the characteristics of biological samples, such as the eye lens, body hair, and skin cancers,[16] the application of Ps lifetime to medicine has not been realized yet. Recently, a prototype PET system was used to measure the o-Ps lifetime of cardiac myxomas and adipose tissues extracted from a human body, and their o-Ps lifetime imaging was demonstrated.[17] The feasibility for the Ps lifetime to add new information about the electron density in vivo to PET images has begun to be seen as a reasonable expectation.

As one of the possible medical applications, sensing of the oxygen partial pressure in living tissue was pointed out.[10] The o-Ps lifetimes were measured for three ^{22}Na solutions with different dissolved oxygen concentrations. The respective oxygen partial pressures pO$_2$ were 0 mm Hg (N$_2$-saturated), 159 mm Hg (air-saturated), and 750 mm Hg (O$_2$-saturated). The radioactivity was

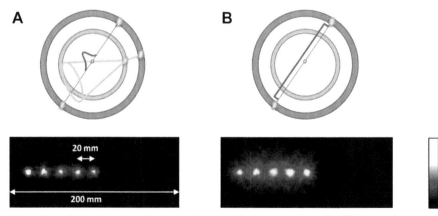

Fig. 6. Demonstration of the reconstruction-less β^+-γ coincidence imaging with a ^{44}Sc point-like source measured at offsets from center to 80 mm with 20 mm steps and all summed (*A*) compared with simple LOR backprojection image (*B*). The transaxial slices are displayed.

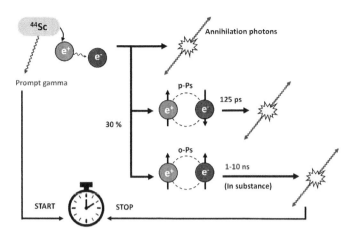

190 kBq for each. The counts obtained were 49 million for the N_2-saturated solution, 59 million for the air-saturated solution, and 43 million for the O_2-saturated solution. The o-Ps lifetime values were calculated from the detection time difference histogram, and o-Ps annihilation rates (inverse of the o-Ps lifetime) [μs^{-1}] were obtained. A linearity was found in **Fig. 8** between the oxygen concentration and the Ps annihilation rate. The linearity comes from the fact that the chance for o-Ps to meet with O_2 is proportional to pO_2. The equation to calculate the oxygen partial pressure pO_2 [mm Hg] from the o-Ps annihilation rate Γ [μs^{-1}] was expressed as follows:

$$pO_2 = 26.3(1.1) \times [\Gamma - 519.9(1.6)] \qquad (4)$$

The number in each set of parentheses is the uncertainty (1σ) calculated from the number of counts. Based on the uncertainty, the sensitivity, that is, pO_2 resolution, was estimated to be *ca.* 10 mm Hg when 300 million counts are obtained in the ROI and to be *ca.* 5 mm Hg when 1 billion counts are obtained. The pO_2 of healthy liver tissue

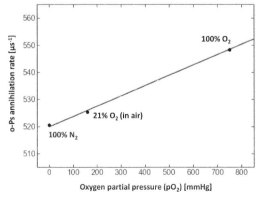

Fig. 8. Linearity between the oxygen concentration (pO_2) and the o-Ps annihilation rate.

cells is reported to be *ca.* 41 mm Hg,[18] and that of liver tumor cells to be *ca.* 6 mm Hg.[19] Assuming that they can be distinguished when the difference is more than twice the resolution (1σ), the required resolution was 17 mm Hg. The experimental result suggested that pO_2 imaging by the o-Ps lifetime has enough sensitivity in living tissue.

To obtain Ps lifetime images using PET, triple coincidence of the prompt gamma ray and 511 keV annihilation photon pair in a single decay event is required. The WGI prototype achieved a positional accuracy of approximately 6.7 mm for [44]Sc reconstruction-less imaging at the triple coincidence.[7] Conventional time-of-flight (TOF)-PET systems that identify the detection time difference of the 511 keV annihilation photon pair can also localize the source position. A state-of-the-art TOF-PET system with a 214-picosecond timing resolution[20] translates into a positional accuracy of about 3 cm. WGI reconstruction-less imaging has a potential to obtain o-Ps lifetime images more accurately.

In a practical scenario for medical applications, it is necessary to periodically calibrate the accuracy of the obtained o-Ps lifetime in some way. Although there have been several articles describing o-Ps lifetimes in various tissues of the living body,[21] less has been discussed about the accuracy of these lifetimes. Therefore, using certified reference materials with known Ps lifetimes,[22] the o-Ps lifetime values were validated in a 2D Ps lifetime image.[23] Two TOF-PET detectors with a 250-picosecond timing resolution were oppositely placed each other (**Fig. 9A**). Two thin-film [22]Na sources were individually sandwiched between 2 types of certified reference materials having known o-Ps lifetimes of 2.1 nanoseconds and 1.62 nanoseconds that were then placed between the detectors and measured for 1 hour. Triple coincidence events were extracted from the measurement

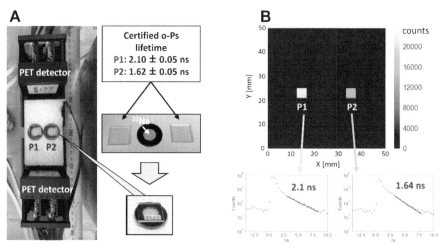

Fig. 9. (*A*) Experimental setup for the 2D o-Ps lifetime imaging. (*B*) Two-dimensional activity distribution and obtained detection time difference histograms. The calculated o-Ps lifetimes are also shown.

data, and detection time difference histograms at points P1 and P2 were obtained from the 2D projection image (**Fig. 9**B). The o-Ps lifetime value of each point was calculated and both were close to the certified values. The result represents the first demonstration that the accuracy of o-Ps lifetime imaging could be verified by using substances traceable to metrology standards.

ANIMAL IMAGING AND POTENTIAL CLINICAL APPLICATIONS

Gamma rays are the only way to transmit information from deep within a living human body to external detectors. Therefore, PET is widely used in various clinical settings; however, PET can detect only pairs of annihilation radiation. A combined Compton and PET system is expected to be used for medical purposes by detecting single gamma rays as well as pairs of annihilation radiation, potentially expanding the choice of radionuclides used in in vivo imaging and improving the image quality. For example, using a Compton-PET system with ^{89}Zr, which emits 4 times more 909-keV gamma rays than positrons, could have a potential to improve the image quality.

^{89}Zr has been intensively used in medical and biological research. This is probably due to the increased availability of monoclonal antibodies and their stable chelation with metallic radionuclides.[24,25] Although ^{18}F-fluorodeoxyglucose (FDG) is the first choice for detecting malignant tumors by imaging regional glucose metabolism, tumor subtypes or specific characteristics are difficult to be identified by ^{18}F-FDG PET. Generally, ^{18}F-FDG accumulates more intensively in tumors with higher malignancy. Contrarily, most tumors

expressing a specific receptor or antigen are differentiated-types of tumors, namely with low-grade malignancy, therefore such tumors frequently show low ^{18}F-FDG accumulation. The combination of imaging both the regional glucose metabolism and the distribution of specific receptors or antigens can help in the assessment of the details of tumors. Furthermore, imaging the distribution of specific immune cells within tumors as well as surrounding them can help in prediction of the effect of treatment by immune checkpoint inhibitors.[26,27]

One of the candidates among malignant tumors that effectively benefits from the Compton-PET system using ^{89}Zr-labeled antibody is multiple myeloma. Multiple myeloma is a tumor of plasma cells, which have pivotal roles in the adaptive immune response. After suffering from an infection, a person becomes immune to the same infection due to the secretion of specific antibodies by plasma cells. Patients with multiple myeloma are highly susceptible to recurrent infection and suffer from multiple-organ dysfunctions caused by the oversecreted abnormal antibodies from the malignant plasma cells. Complete cures for multiple myeloma are challenging but a specific antigen on tumor cells has now become a target of imaging as well as treatment. No detectable tumor cells after treatment suggest a favorable prognosis, which is described as minimal residual disease-negative.[28] The next issue that researchers should address is how to detect the residual tumor cells.

A Compton-PET system with ^{89}Zr is expected to be able to evaluate residual tumors. A small animal imaging experiment was conducted with multiple myeloma using the WGI prototype. After 3-Gy gamma ray irradiation, a severe combined

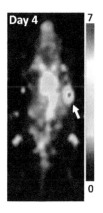 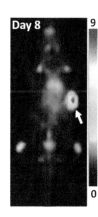 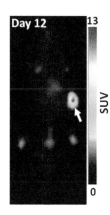

Fig. 10. MIP images of a tumor-burdened SICD mouse measured by the WGI prototype. [89]Zr-anti-CD38 antibody was significantly accumulated in the tumor (*arrows*).

immunodeficiency (SICD) mouse was implanted subcutaneously in the right flank with 3×10^7 RPMI8226 cells in 100 μL of phosphate-buffered saline. On day 12 after the implantation, the tumor volume reached approximately 180 mm³. As an agent for imaging, anti-CD38 antibody (daratumumab) conjugated to [89]Zr through a chelator (deferoxamine). The [89]Zr-daratumumab at the dose of 3.3 MBq was injected via a tail vein. WGI imaging was performed on days 4, 8, and 12 after [89]Zr-daratumumab injection. After WGI imaging on day 12, the mouse was euthanized for ex vivo biodistribution analysis. Tumor, blood, liver, and other organs were sampled, their weight and radioactivity were measured, and %ID/g values were calculated. WGI imaging showed that [89]Zr-daratumumab uptake in tumors increased over time, reaching to the standardized uptake value 9.8 on day 12 (**Fig.10**). The uptake in the healthy tissues gradually decreased with time except for the bone joints. Respective %ID/g values of tumor, blood, and liver were 0.70, 0.12, and 0.04, respectively. It was estimated that [89]Zr-daratumumab accumulated in RPMI8226 tumor cells at approximately 730 fmol/mg. Although this was a preliminary result, it showed that WGI can provide quantitative values about the amount of antigen expression of a tumor. From this, it is believed that WGI is helpful to define the minimal residual disease based on a quantitative value obtained noninvasively.

As shown in **Fig.10**, images at a late time point such as day12 after the tracer injection can be obtained. This advantage is due to the long half-life of [89]Zr (~78.4 hours) and the high sensitivity of WGI. Radiolabeled antibody distributions typically take a longer time to reach equilibrium to be scanned, which is opposite the behavior in imaging of regional blood flow rates, glucose metabolism rates, or receptor densities. Therefore, WGI can be more helpful than PET for imaging tumors that appear clearly at a late time point by [89]Zr-antibodies.[29]

Other applications using WGI could be for in vivo cell tracking. Jacob and colleagues[30] reported the feasibility of [89]Zr-labeled regulatory T cell tracking using PET. The anti-inflammatory effect of T cells is expected to be applied in treatment of inflammatory diseases caused by autoimmune disorders or chronic reactions to transplanted organs. To evaluate the efficacy, localization and quantification of regulatory T cells are needed. They also pointed out that radioactivity higher than 0.3 Bq per cell can impairs the viability of the T cells themselves. Therefore, T cells should be labeled with low-dose [89]Zr to image immune cells. It is also expected that WGI will be helpful in tracking radiosensitive cells such as immune cells.

WGI has the additional potential of pO_2 mm Hg imaging by measuring the Ps lifetime. In oncology, hypoxic malignant tumors are resistant to various treatments. Although PET imaging using ^{18}F-fluoromisonidazoel and ^{18}F-fluoroazomycinarabionofuranoside (FAZA) are helpful to identify hypoxic areas in tumors, the quantitative value depends on relative ratios, where tumor-to-muscle is commonly used. An absolute value, namely pO_2 mm Hg, is needed to decide the treatment intensity based on the data from many patients with the same type tumor.

SUMMARY

In clinical practice, generally speaking, it is essential to use as many as possible individual clinical data for accurate diagnosis. In nuclear medicine, this concept would be realized by using as many as possible detectable gamma rays for imaging—this is WGI. The use of unusual positron emitters such as [89]Zr and [44]Sc with WGI is expected to break through current limitations in nuclear medicine. Although 909-keV gamma rays emitted from [89]Zr are only a source of noise in PET, they can be used as a signal in WGI. [89]Zr-WGI may enable earlier detection of a small amount of tumor cells such as multiple myeloma. The time difference between positron emission and the third gamma emission is almost zero in ^{44}Sc, and this characteristic may lead to novel reconstruction-less imaging as well as Ps lifetime imaging, which may realize quantitative hypoxia tumor imaging.

ACKNOWLEDGMENTS

The authors would like to thank Dr Eiji Yoshida, Dr Kotaro Nagatsu, Dr Kengo Shibuya, Prof Katia Parodi, Prof Yoichi Imai, Dr Mariko Ishibashi, and Dr Atsushi B Tsuji for development of WGI and its application. The authors also would like to thank the following funding sources: the Japan Society for the Promotion of Science, Japan (JSPS) KAKENHI Grants (20H05667, 21K19936 and 22K12881), the QST President Grants and the Nakatani Foundation, Japan.

DISCLOSURE

The authors have nothing to disclose.

REFERENCES

1. Zaidi H, Koral KF. Scatter modelling and compensation in emission tomography. Eur J Nucl Med Mol Imag 2004;31:761–82.
2. Hutton BF, Buvat I, Beekman FJ. Review and current status of SPECT scatter correction. Phys Med Biol 2011;56:R85–112.
3. Llosá G. Rafecas M Hybrid PET/Compton-camera imaging: an imager for the next generation. Eur Phys J Plus 2023;138:214.
4. Todd RW, Nightingale JM, Everett DB. A proposed γ camera. Nature 1974;251:132–4.
5. Tashima H, Yamaya T. Compton imaging for medical applications. Radiol Phys Technol 2022;15:187–205.
6. Nakano T, Sakai M, Torikai K, et al. Imaging of ^{99m}Tc-DMSA and ^{18}F-FDG in humans using a Si/CdTe Compton camera. Phys Med Biol 2020;65:05LT01.
7. Yoshida E, Tashima H, Nagatsu K, et al. Whole gamma imaging: a new concept of PET combined with Compton imaging. Phys Med Biol 2020;65:125013.
8. Tashima H, Yoshida E, Wakizaka H, et al. 3D Compton image reconstruction method for whole gamma imaging. Phys Med Biol 2020;65:225038.
9. Moskal P, Jasińska B, Stępień EŁ, et al. Positronium in medicine and biology. Nature Reviews Physics 2019;1:527–9.
10. Shibuya K, Saito H, Nishikido F, et al. Oxygen sensing ability of positronium atom for tumor hypoxia imaging. Commun Phys 2020;3:173.
11. Shimura N, Kamada K, Gunji A, et al. Zr doped GSO:Ce single crystals and their scintillation performance. IEEE Symp Conf Rec Nucl Sci 2004;2720–3.
12. Hirano Y, Nitta M, Inadama N, et al. Performance evaluation of a depth-of-interaction detector by use of position-sensitive PMT with a super-bialkali photocathode. Radiol Phys Technol 2013;7:57–66.
13. Kamada K, Yanagida T, Pejchal J, et al. Crystal growth and scintillation properties of Ce doped $Gd_3(Ga,Al)_5O_{12}$ single crystals. IEEE Trans Nucl Sci 2012;59:2112–5.
14. Tashima H, Yoshida E, Wakizaka H, et al. Development of a hybrid image reconstruction algorithm combining PET and Compton events for whole gamma imaging. Boston, MA, USA: IEEE nuclear science Symposium and medical imaging conference (NSS/MIC); 2020. p. 1–2. https://doi.org/10.1109/NSS/MIC42677.2020.9507841.
15. Sitarz M, Cussonneau J-P, Matulewicz, et al. Radionuclide candidates for β+γ coincidence PET: an overview. Appl Radiat Isot 2020;155:108898.
16. Chen H, Van Horn DJ, Jean YC. Applications of positron annihilation spectroscopy to life science. Defect Diffusion Forum 2012;331:275–93.
17. Moskal P, Dulski K, Chug N, et al. Positronium imaging with the novel multiphoton PET scanner. Sci Adv 2021;7:1–10.
18. Carreau A, El Hafny-Rahbi B, Matejuk A, et al. Why is the partial oxygen pressure of human tissues a crucial parameter? Small molecules and hypoxia. J Cell Mol Med 2011;15:1239–53.
19. Vaupel P, Höckel M, Mayer A. Detection and characterization of tumor hypoxia using pO_2 histography. Antioxidants Redox Signal 2007;9:1221–35.
20. Van Sluis JJ, De Jong J, Schaar J, et al. Performance characteristics of the digital biograph vision PET/CT system. J Nucl Med 2019;60:1031–6.
21. Bass SD, Mariazz S, Moskal P, et al. Positronium Physics and Biomedical Applications, https://doi.org/10.48550/arXiv.2302.09246
22. Ito K, Oka T, Kobayashi Y, et al. Interlaboratory comparison of positron annihilation lifetime measurements for synthetic fused silica and polycarbonate. J Appl Phys 2008;104:026102.
23. Takyu S, Shibuya K, Nishikido F, et al. Two-dimensional positronium lifetime imaging using certified reference materials. Appl Phys Express 2022;15:106001.
24. van Dongen GAMS, Beaino W, Windhorst AD, et al. The role of ^{89}Zr-Immuno-PET in navigating and de-risking the development of biopharmaceuticals. J Nucl Med 2021;62:438–45.
25. Chomet M, Schreurs M, Bolijn MJ, et al. Head-to-head comparison of DFO* and DFO chelators: selection of the best candidate for clinical 89Zr-immuno-PET. Eur J Nucl Med Mol Imag 2021;48:694–707.
26. van den Ende T, van den Boorn HG, Hoonhout NM, et al. Priming the tumor immune microenvironment with chemo(radio)therapy: a systematic review

across tumor types. Biochim Biophys Acta Rev Cancer 2020;1874:188386.

27. Niemeijer AN, Leung D, Huisman MC, et al. Whole body PD-1 and PD-L1 positron emission tomography in patients with non-small-cell lung cancer. Nat Commun 2018;9(1):4664.

28. Paiva B, van Dongen JJ. Orfao A New criteria for response assessment: role of minimal residual disease in multiple myeloma. Blood 2015;125:3059–68.

29. Rosar F, Schaefer-Schuler A, Bartholomä M, et al. [^{89}Zr]Zr-PSMA-617 PET/CT in biochemical recurrence of prostate cancer: first clinical experience from a pilot study including biodistribution and dose estimates. Eur J Nucl Med Mol Imag 2022;49:4736–47.

30. Jacob J, Volpe A, Peng Q, et al. Radiolabelling of polyclonally expanded human regulatory T cells (Treg) with ^{89}Zr-oxine for medium-Term in vivo cell tracking. Molecules 2023;28:1482.

Transforming Neurology and Psychiatry
Organ-specific PET Instrumentation and Clinical Applications

Ahmed Taha, MD[a,1], Amer Alassi, MD[a,1], Albert Gjedde, MD, DSc[b,c], Dean F. Wong, MD, PhD[d,2,*]

KEYWORDS

- PET - Brain energy metabolism - Neurochemistry - Neuroreceptors

KEY POINTS

- PET identifies changes in brain function and metabolism at early stages of neuropsychiatric disorders, even before the onset of clinical symptoms, potentially leading to earlier interventions and better outcomes.
- PET distinguishes different neurologic and psychiatric disorders with overlapping clinical symptoms, such as AD, PD, and frontotemporal dementia, by visualizing distinct patterns of brain metabolism and function.
- PET helps identify the extent of tumor involvement, differentiate between tumor recurrence and treatment-related changes (eg, radiation necrosis), and assess the response to treatments such as chemotherapy and radiotherapy. Furthermore, PET imaging can provide insights into tumor biology and metabolism, which can guide the selection of targeted therapies and personalized treatment strategies.
- PET monitors the effectiveness of treatments in neurologic and psychiatric disorders, such as evaluating the response to medications in epilepsy or measuring the changes in brain metabolism after pharmacologic or behavioural interventions in depression.
- PET assesses target engagement and receptor-mediated mechanisms of drugs in neurologic and psychiatric disorders. It visualizes drug-target interaction, optimizing dosing strategies, rationalizing drug treatments, and facilitating personalized medicine approaches.
- PET serves as a complementary tool alongside other neuroimaging techniques, such as MRI and CT scans, to provide a comprehensive understanding of the underlying pathophysiology and to guide clinical decision-making.
- PET has limits by its cost, availability, lack of FDA approval for clinical use, and the need for exposure to ionizing radiation. It may not be suitable for all patients or as a firstline diagnostic tool in all cases.

[a] Mallinckrodt Institute of Radiology, Washington University in St Louis, Saint Louis, MO, USA; [b] Department of Clinical Medicine, Translational Neuropsychiatry Unit, Aarhus University, Denmark; [c] Department of Neuroscience, University of Copenhagen, Denmark; [d] Mallinckrodt Institute of Radiology, Departments of Radiology, Psychiatry, Neurology, Neuroscience, Washington University in St Louis, Saint Louis, MO, USA
[1] Shared first authorship.
[2] Senior author.
* Corresponding author. Mallinckrodt Institute of Radiology, Washington University in St Louis, 4525 Scott Avenue, Campus Box 8225, Saint Louis, MO 63110.
E-mail address: dfwong@wustl.edu

PET Clin 19 (2024) 95–103
https://doi.org/10.1016/j.cpet.2023.06.002
1556-8598/24/© 2023 Elsevier Inc. All rights reserved.

INTRODUCTION

In neurology and psychiatry, recent advances by PET have yielded unprecedented insights into the functioning of the human brain and the development of novel treatment strategies.[1,2] The introduction of 2-[18F]fluoro-2-deoxy-D-glucose (FDG) from 2-[11C]deoxyglucose in 1976 represented a great leap forward.[3] The development revolutionized brain PET imaging[4] by means of FDG that evolved into one of the most commonly used radiotracers.[5]

High-Resolution PET Devices for Neuroimaging

The first PET devices that served brain imaging paved the way for the current understanding of brain function and disease. Dedicated brain PET devices such as the high-resolution research tomograph (HRRT)[6] and new devices such as PET brain hemisphere imaging[7] resulted in high-resolution PET images that offered improved spatial resolution. Greater resolution allowed visualization of brain structures and functions with a greater precision that approached the theoretic limit. The enhanced resolution facilitates the detection of subtle abnormalities of brain function that can be critical for the diagnosis and monitoring of specific neurologic and psychiatric disorders.

Integration of PET with MRI and Computed Tomography

Hybrid modalities, such as PET/computed tomography (CT)[8] and PET/MRI,[9] provide better accuracy, higher quality functional information, and superior soft tissue contrast. The need for more accurate, reliable, and reproducible diagnostic and prognostic information, especially from PET brain imaging of neurodegenerative diseases, shifted the analysis from qualitative visual interpretation to quantitative analysis.[10] Users now pursue quantification to address the inherent issues associated with qualitative assessment of PET imaging, including inter-reader variability,[11] limited sensitivity to delicate variations,[12] and dependence on image quality.[13]

Novel Radiotracers for Improved Specificity

New radiotracers enable visualization of molecular targets in the brain, revealing insights into key processes underlying specific neurologic and psychiatric disorders and aiding development of targeted treatments.

CLINICAL APPLICATIONS IN NEUROLOGY
Alzheimer Disease

Early brain imaging of Alzheimer disease (AD) used FDG that recently attracted renewed interest as a direct marker of cortical functionality in keeping with the recent AT(N) proposal.[14–16] Later visualization of AD's hallmarks, that is, accumulation of extracellular amyloid beta (Aβ), and intracellular neurofibrillary tau tangles, enabled the early diagnosis of AD.[17] Early diagnosis allows for timely intervention that may slow disease progression. Postmortem pathologic studies[14] mostly underwent replacement by the introduction of the in vivo imaging of Aβ by means of the Pittsburgh compound B[18] and the approval of 3 F-18 amyloid tracers, florbetapir,[19] florbetaben,[20] and flutemetamol.[21] As for tau tangles, multiple generations of tau tracers now exist, with each new generation improving the pharmacokinetics, specificity, and selectivity.[22] Tau tracers include first-generation THK compounds (eg,.THK-523),[23] the second-generation tracer AV-1451 (flortaucipir, T807),[24] and third-generation tracers such as PI-2620,[25] MK-6240,[26] GTP-1,[27] and RO-948.[28,29] The latter was promising in showing regional uptake in subjects with AD (**Fig. 1**).

Multiple methods serve PET image quantification in AD,[30] including the standardized uptake value ratio (SUVr).[31] Despite the lack of full quantitation, SUVr is popular because of its clinical simplicity, compared with more complex and demanding quantitative techniques that require arterial blood sampling or reference tissue quantification and other requirements.[30] The Centiloid scale is a recently introduced method of universal amyloid PET quantification that allows more uniform comparisons of amyloid accumulation results across different PET centers and different amyloid PET tracers.[30]

Parkinson Disease

In Parkinson disease (PD) and other synuclein neuropathies, the hallmark is abnormal alpha-synuclein (α-syn) deposition.[32] In contrast to AD, the development of a radiotracer for this group of diseases is more challenging, because of a much lower concentration of α-syn aggregates in the brain compared with Aβ or tau,[33] poor understanding of the binding mechanism,[34] and obstacles facing the translation of new α-syn PET tracers to clinical research, mainly because of the in vivo versus in vitro structural heterogeneity of brain-derived material from patients with PD in vivo.[35] In initial studies, tracers such as the cocaine congener [11C]Win35,428 revealed MPTP-induced activity reductions in primates and later in PD.[36] Multiple PET tracers for α-synuclein neuropathies exist, including the standard [18F]FDOPA tracer of the activity of aromatic L-amino acid decarboxylase, the key enzyme involved in the

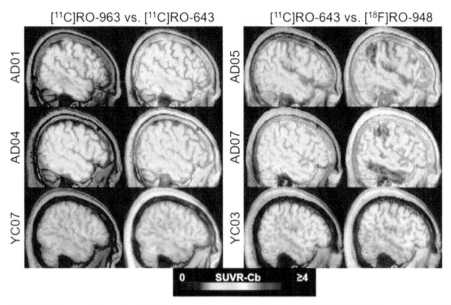

Fig. 1. Sagittal SUVR images from the first human evaluation of 11C-RO-963, 11C-RO-643, and 18F-RO-948 radioligands, applied to same subjects with AD and young controls (YCs). The regional retention of 18F- RO-948 seemed to distinguish between subjects with AD and YCs. Cerebellar cortex (Cb) YC AD subject IDs: AD01, AD02, AD05, and AD07 and YC IDs: YC07 and YC03. (This research was originally published in JNM. Dean F. Wong et al. Characterization of 3 Novel Tau Radiopharmaceuticals, 11C-RO-963, 11C-RO-643, and 18F-RO-948, in Healthy Controls and in Alzheimer Subjects. Journal of Nuclear Medicine Dec 2018, 59 (12) 1869-1876. © SNMMI.)

synthesis of dopamine.[37] Other tracers including [11C]CFT (a.k.a. Win 35,428) and [11C]DTBZ reveal the density of nigrostriatal dopaminergic terminals affected in PD.[38] Standard [18F]FDG mainly identifies characteristic patterns of hypometabolism in patients with PD or other parkinsonian syndromes.[39] Tracers such as [11C]PK11195 and [18F]DPA-714 serve to study the role of inflammation in PD.[40] The tracers [11C]PBB3 and [18F]PM-PBB3 reveal tau protein aggregates in progressive supranuclear palsy and in other atypical parkinsonian syndromes.[41]

Understanding the Pathophysiology of Epilepsy and Other Neurologic Disorders

PET imaging contributed to mapping of frontotemporal dementia with FDG[42] and microglia activation in traumatic brain injury with [11C]PK11195.[43] Recently, the Food and Drug Administration (FDA) approved the striatal dopamine transporter visualization by DATSCAN ([123I]lioflupane injection) as the first single-photon emission computed tomography (SPECT) imaging of patients with dementia with Lewy bodies, years after the federal agency approved the same tracer for the imaging of patients with suspected PD.[44] FDG-PET has been deemed useful to the diagnosis, evaluation, and planning of surgery for patients with epilepsy by identifying the seizure focus as crucial to the planning of surgery of patients with refractory epilepsy.

FDG-PET plays a significant complementary role to methods such as MRI and electroencephalography (EEG),[45] in the localization of seizure foci in temporal and extratemporal lobes.[46]

Neurooncology and Brain Death

PET is essential to the imaging of brain tumors that provides insights beyond MRI. PET yields differential diagnosis, grading, and delineating tumor involvement for surgery and radiotherapy planning. PET is also used for monitoring and posttreatment prognostics. PET radiotracers have advantages to MRI because of the insensitivity to blood-brain barrier (BBB) disruption, remaining unaffected except for disease-specific pathophysiologic mechanisms, unlike contrast-enhanced MRI.[47]

Glioma

Tracer [18F]FDG can identify high-grade gliomas.[48] Low-grade gliomas (of the World Health Organization [WHO] grades I and II) typically reveal uptake similar to white matter. High-grade tumors (WHO grade III) may be difficult to distinguish from the background activity of gray matter, unlike grade IV tumors (glioblastoma multiforme) that generally show tracer uptake above the gray-matter background. PET by [18F]FDG also directs biopsy attempts to the most aggressive regions of a lesion.[49] Although [18F]FDG is of prognostic value in high-grade gliomas,[48] it is of limited value to treatment planning. With 90% sensitivity and specificity, amino acid PET may help differentiate gliomas from nonneoplastic tissue,[50] but a small proportion of gliomas show no amino acid uptake at all,[51] and some inflammation cases are reported to have only moderate amino acid uptake.[52]

Meningioma

Somatostatin receptor (SSTR) ligands are the radiotracers of choice, as meningiomas almost invariably express the SSTR type 2 receptor.[53] PET with SSTR ligands discriminates well between meningioma accumulation and other tissue entities, including chronic inflammation.[54] PET with SSTR ligands also is useful in cases of ambiguous, noncontributive MRI or uptake in specific regions that are difficult to identify by MRI, such as the base of the skull and bony structures.[47]

Primary central nervous system lymphoma

[18F]FDG assists the diagnostic task by differentiating primary central nervous system (CNS) lymphomas from other malignant brain tumors such as glioblastomas and metastases.[47] At the time of initial diagnosis, differentiation between primary CNS lymphomas and infectious lesions is also possible with PET by [18F]FDG of immunocompromised patients.[55] However, to date no study revealed a significant impact of PET results on the overall survival of patients with primary CNS lymphoma.[47]

Brain metastases

Irrespective of the primary cancer, PET by [18F]FDG or amino acid tracers is recommended for the differential diagnosis of recurrent brain metastases and radiation-induced changes. PET with amino acids seems to be superior to [18F]FDG PET and perfusion or diffusion-weighted MRI for the differential diagnosis of radionecrosis and recurrent brain metastases.[56] The differential diagnosis of brain metastases from malignant brain tumors nevertheless is challenging with the use of PET imaging, because PET by [18F]FDG has highly positive results in brain metastases and glioblastomas,[57] with brain metastases exhibiting similar levels of expression of the L-amino-acid transporters as gliomas.[58]

Experimental PET in oncology

Other experimental PET radiopharmaceuticals serve to assess aspects of tumor cellular activity other than glucose metabolism. The evaluation of DNA synthesis with [18F]fluorothymidine is useful in patients with aggressive, enhancing tumors, where the BBB has disintegrated. However, thymidine metabolism is complex, and amino acid agents have potentially high specificity and

sensitivity, even in lower-grade tumors and in lesions where the BBB remains intact. The agents include [11C]methionine, [18F]fluorodopa, and [18F]fluoroethyltyrosine.[49]

Brain death

PET serves to differentiate vegetative or unresponsive wakefulness syndrome from the minimally conscious state.[59] Accuracy and speed in making the diagnosis of brain death become critical when organ donation is considered, and life support systems are in demand. Although the diagnosis of brain death is clinical, the diagnosis may be difficult. Although confirmatory ancillary tests (such as EEG) may increase certainty, they cannot themselves establish the diagnosis of brain death.[60] In brain death, pressure increases due to edema, softening, necrosis, and autolysis, hindering intracranial perfusion beyond internal carotid arteries. Radionuclide brain death study is a noninvasive alternative to catheter angiography, useful for equivocal EEG and clinical criteria or when urgent decisions must be made. The study is not affected by drug intoxication or hypothermia, and an abnormal radionuclide angiogram showing no cerebral perfusion is more specific than an isoelectric EEG for brain death. The [99mTc]-labeled radiopharmaceuticals assess dynamic flow, with [99mTc]HMPAO and [99mTc]ECD studies preferred over [99mTc]DTPA due to easy interpretation relying only on delayed images. Because tracer uptake by living brain cells requires intact blood flow, cerebral uptake is absent without flow. Tracer [99mTc]HMPAO is injected intravenously, and delayed bedside planar imaging suffices, without need for flow images or SPECT. Brain death is indicated by lack of brain visualization by [99mTc]HMPAO due to limited flow to the skull base. Although not used alone for diagnosis, MRI techniques provide supportive evidence in proper clinical settings of intracerebral blood flow presence. Repeat studies may be necessary for severely decreased but not completely absent perfusion.

CLINICAL APPLICATIONS IN PSYCHIATRY

PET makes the study of the neurobiology of psychiatric disorders possible,[61] providing insight into underlying brain mechanisms under different conditions. Here, we briefly mention selected disorders, including major depressive disorder, bipolar mood disorder, schizophrenia, and substance use disorder.

Major Depressive Disorder

PET imaging reveals alterations of brain metabolism and neurotransmissions by transmitters such as norepinephrine, serotonin, and dopamine. In individuals with major depressive disorder (MDD), tracer studies expand the understanding of the underlying pathology and provide guidance toward treatment selection. PET studies have demonstrated reduced serotonin transporter availability in the brains of patients with MDD, which may contribute to the pathophysiology of the disorder.[62] Interestingly, patients suffering from a depressive episode show overall increased cerebral serotonin transporter availability as symptoms decline.[63] Studies of MDD with radiolabeled dopamine $D_{2/3}$ receptor agonists revealed higher $D_{2/3}$ receptor availability in ventral striatum together with greater anhedonia.[64] Also, results from PET imaging suggest a potential link between inflammation and MDD.[65]

Bipolar Mood Disorder

Investigations include the roles of dopamine, serotonin, and glutamate transmitter systems, as well as changes of brain glucose metabolism. In one study, researchers investigated the effects of treatment with a glucagon-like peptide-1 receptor agonist on brain structure and function in individuals with mood disorders that included bipolar disorder. PET images recorded changes of brain glucose metabolism, and the results revealed weight loss–related changes in frontostriatal brain structures.[66] In another study, the investigators investigated the relationship between cerebral glutamate levels and the severity of mood symptoms in patients with (Bipolar Mood Disorder) BP, and the findings revealed a positive correlation between glutamate levels and symptom severity, suggesting that glutamatergic dysfunction plays a role in the pathophysiology of bipolar disorder.[67]

Schizophrenia

In schizophrenia, PET imaging elucidated abnormalities of dopamine and glutamate neurotransmission.[68] Findings by PET shed light on the pathophysiology of schizophrenia,[69] and the findings informed the development of novel antipsychotic medications that target specific neurotransmitter systems.[70] In a study, the investigators examined the relationship between glutamate levels in the anterior cingulate cortex and clinical outcomes in patients with first-episode schizophrenia following treatment. The findings revealed that lower baseline glutamate levels were associated with a better clinical response to treatment, suggesting that glutamatergic dysfunction[71] may play a role in the pathophysiology of schizophrenia and treatment response.[72] In a different study, the researchers discussed the role of serotonin receptors in schizophrenia, highlighting the potential of PET imaging to provide insights into the neurobiology of schizophrenia, particularly regarding the neurotransmitter serotonin's involvement in the disorder.[73]

Substance Use Disorder

PET imaging extensively has been used to study the neurobiological underpinnings of substance use disorder,[74] especially regarding the role of neurotransmitters such as the opioid systems, in the development and maintenance of addiction. Investigations focused on relations of depressive symptoms and peripheral dopamine transporter (DAT) methylation to neural reactivity to alcohol cues in alcohol use disorder. The results demonstrated an association between increased DAT methylation, depressive symptoms, and the reactivity to the cues that suggested that PET images provide insights into the interaction between depression and addiction.[75] Assessing dopamine $D_{2/3}$ receptor availability in methamphetamine users and examining the relationship to impulsivity and risk-taking behaviors showed that lower $D_{2/3}$ receptor availability in the striatum is associated with increased impulsivity and risk taking, highlighting the role of the dopaminergic system in the development and maintenance of methamphetamine use disorder.[75]

Strengths and Limitations of Using PET Imaging in Neuropsychiatric Disorders

PET has the unique ability to visualize molecular processes in vivo. Its wide applicability, and the fact that PET tracers target different molecules and receptors, allow for the study of specific aspects of brain function, including metabolism, neurotransmitter release, and inflammation. On the other hand, PET imaging is expensive and requires access to specialized equipment, including cyclotrons and radiochemistry facilities. Furthermore, PET imaging involves exposure to ionizing radiation that may limit the frequency of imaging sessions and the use of PET in certain populations, such as pregnant women and children. Some PET tracers lack specificity that may generate false-positive or false-negative findings. PET imaging also has relatively low temporal resolution compared with other neuroimaging techniques, such as EEG or magnetoencephalography.[76]

PET NEURORECEPTOR IMAGING AS AN AID TO EARLY THERAPEUTIC DRUG DEVELOPMENT

The imaging of dopamine receptors and the quantification of receptor number and affinity depend on receptor occupancy (now known as target engagement).[77] This measure has been used in the development of almost all FDA-approved antipsychotics (with some dopamine receptor activity) and antidepressants (especially serotonin reuptake inhibitors). Preclinical and early phase 1 studies of healthy volunteers have guided dose selection of the therapeutic drug for future use in the intended patient population.[78] This principle now has undergone expansion to many studies, primarily of drugs used in neurology such as those applied to movement disorders with glutamate receptor activity.

THE ROLE OF DEDICATED BRAIN SCANNER AND ITS UNIQUE APPLICATIONS TO ASSESS CENTRAL NERVOUS SYSTEM DISORDERS

The development of dedicated brain PET hardware was initially motivated by the need for improved performance compared with whole-body devices, specifically better spatial resolution, or higher sensitivity to enable the imaging of small brain structures.[79] Within the EXPLORER consortium, the construction of the world's first total-body PET/CT scanner was completed. Regarding brain imaging, there was excellent delineation of the smaller structures of the brain, with the high sensitivity of the scanner supporting a very-high-resolution reconstruction without incurring a high noise penalty, even at low injected dose (80 MBq).[80] Many conventional stand-alone PET scanners have been developed. The best-known dedicated brain PET scanner is the HRRT built by CTI PET Systems, Inc (Knoxville, TN, USA).[81-83] A next-generation ultra-high-performance human brain PET, the NeuroEXPLORER, has been designed showing dramatic sensitivity increase compared with the HRRT that reliably allows measuring uptake in small nuclei and opening new frontiers of imaging neurotransmitter dynamics.[84]

Several unconventional scanner geometries increased the sensitivity by using detectors arranged in a compact hemisphere resembling a helmet, which improved the solid-angle coverage at most cortical brain structures and the cerebellum.[85] Substantial progress has been made in the field of dedicated brain PET instrumentation. However, sustained effort is still needed to design specialized products that can broaden our understanding of the human brain and address clinical needs in neurology and psychiatry.[79]

FUTURE PERSPECTIVES AND CONCLUSION

PET technology has immense potential for furthering understanding of the brain and associated disorders, including advancements in high-resolution tomographs and hybrid imaging modalities. Novel radiotracers targeting specific neurotransmitter systems and molecular markers provide opportunities to unveil intricate mechanisms underlying neurologic and psychiatric conditions. As PET imaging techniques and analysis methods continue to be refined, the field is poised to make significant contributions to personalized medicine for more targeted and effective interventions. PET instrumentation has advanced the fields of neurology and psychiatry, providing insights into pathophysiology and development of effective treatments. Ongoing advancements in PET instrumentation and radiotracer development offer promising prospects for diagnosis and management of these disorders.

FUNDING

Funding NIH PHS grants: R01MH10719705, R21AG062314.

REFERENCES

1. Schöll M, Lockhart SN, Schonhaut DR, et al. PET imaging of tau deposition in the aging human brain. Neuron 2016;89(5):971–82.
2. Schöll M, Damián A, Engler H. Fluorodeoxyglucose PET in neurology and psychiatry. Pet Clin 2014; 9(4):371–90, v.
3. Sokoloff L. The history of neuroscience in autobiography1. Washington, DC Soc: Neurosci; 1996.
4. Noble RM. 18)F-FDG PET/CT brain imaging. J Nucl Med Technol 2021;49(3):215–6.
5. Raichle ME. A brief history of human brain mapping. Trends Neurosci 2009;32(2):118–26.
6. Wienhard K, Schmand M, Casey ME, et al. The ECAT HRRT: performance and first clinical application of the new high resolution research tomograph. IEEE Trans Nucl Sci 2002;49(1):104–10.
7. Takahashi M, Akamatsu G, Iwao Y, et al. Small nuclei identification with a hemispherical brain PET. EJNMMI Physics 2022;9(1):69.
8. Townsend DW. Positron emission tomography/computed tomography. Semin Nucl Med 2008; 38(3):152–66.
9. Pichler BJ, Kolb A, Nägele T, et al. PET/MRI: paving the way for the next generation of clinical multimodality imaging applications. J Nucl Med 2010;51(3):333–6.
10. Carson RE. Pet physiological measurements using constant infusion. Nucl Med Biol 2000;27(7):657–60.
11. Minoshima S, Drzezga AE, Barthel H, et al. SNMMI procedure standard/EANM practice guideline for amyloid PET imaging of the brain 1.0. J Nucl Med 2016;57(8):1316–22.
12. Villemagne VL, Pike KE, Chételat G, et al. Longitudinal assessment of Aβ and cognition in aging and Alzheimer disease. Ann Neurol 2011;69(1):181–92.

13. Kinahan PE, Fletcher JW. Positron emission tomography-computed tomography standardized uptake values in clinical practice and assessing response to therapy. Semin Ultrasound CT MR 2010;31(6):496–505.

14. Jack CR Jr, Bennett DA, Blennow K, et al. NIA-AA Research Framework: toward a biological definition of Alzheimer's disease. Alzheimers Dement 2018; 14(4):535–62.

15. Alavi A, Barrio JR, Werner TJ, et al. Suboptimal validity of amyloid imaging-based diagnosis and management of Alzheimer's disease: why it is time to abandon the approach. Eur J Nucl Med Mol Imag 2019;47(2):225–30.

16. Rischel EB, Gejl M, Brock B, et al. In Alzheimer's disease, amyloid beta accumulation is a protective mechanism that ultimately fails. Alzheimer's Dementia 2022;19(3):771–83.

17. Murphy MP, LeVine H Iii. Alzheimer's disease and the amyloid-β peptide. J Alzheimers Dis 2010;19: 311–23.

18. Klunk WE, Engler H, Nordberg A, et al. Imaging brain amyloid in Alzheimer's disease with Pittsburgh Compound-B. Ann Neurol 2004;55(3):306–19.

19. Wong DF, Rosenberg PB, Zhou Y, et al. In vivo imaging of amyloid deposition in Alzheimer disease using the radioligand 18F-AV-45 (florbetapir [corrected] F 18). J Nucl Med 2010;51(6):913–20.

20. Sabri O, Sabbagh MN, Seibyl J, et al. Florbetaben PET imaging to detect amyloid beta plaques in Alzheimer's disease: phase 3 study. Alzheimer's Dementia 2015;11(8):964–74.

21. Vandenberghe R, Van Laere K, Ivanoiu A, et al. 18F-flutemetamol amyloid imaging in Alzheimer disease and mild cognitive impairment: a phase 2 trial. Ann Neurol 2010;68(3):319–29.

22. Leuzy A, Chiotis K, Lemoine L, et al. Tau PET imaging in neurodegenerative tauopathies—still a challenge. Mol Psychiatr 2019;24(8):1112–34.

23. Fodero-Tavoletti MT, Okamura N, Furumoto S, et al. 18F-THK523: a novel in vivo tau imaging ligand for Alzheimer's disease. Brain 2011;134(Pt 4):1089–100.

24. Chien DT, Szardenings AK, Bahri S, et al. Early clinical PET imaging results with the novel PHF-tau radioligand [F18]-T808. J Alzheimers Dis 2014;38(1): 171–84.

25. Kroth H, Oden F, Molette J, et al. Discovery and preclinical characterization of [(18)F]PI-2620, a next-generation tau PET tracer for the assessment of tau pathology in Alzheimer's disease and other tauopathies. Eur J Nucl Med Mol Imag 2019;46(10):2178–89.

26. Hostetler ED, Walji AM, Zeng Z, et al. Preclinical characterization of 18F-MK-6240, a promising PET tracer for in vivo quantification of human neurofibrillary tangles. J Nucl Med 2016;57(10):1599–606.

27. Sanabria Bohórquez S, Marik J, Ogasawara A, et al. [18 F] GTP1 (Genentech Tau Probe 1), a radioligand for detecting neurofibrillary tangle tau pathology in Alzheimer's disease. Eur J Nucl Med Mol Imag 2019;46:2077–89.

28. Wong DF, Comley RA, Kuwabara H, et al. Characterization of 3 novel tau radiopharmaceuticals, (11)C-RO-963, (11)C-RO-643, and (18)F-RO-948, in healthy controls and in alzheimer subjects. J Nucl Med 2018;59(12): 1869–76.

29. Kuwabara H, Comley RA, Borroni E, et al. Evaluation of (18)F-RO-948 PET for quantitative assessment of tau accumulation in the human brain. J Nucl Med 2018;59(12):1877–84.

30. Pemberton HG, Collij LE, Heeman F, et al. Quantification of amyloid PET for future clinical use: a state-of-the-art review. Eur J Nucl Med Mol Imag 2022;49(10):3508–28.

31. Lopresti BJ, Klunk WE, Mathis CA, et al. Simplified quantification of Pittsburgh Compound B amyloid imaging PET studies: a comparative analysis. J Nucl Med 2005;46(12):1959–72.

32. Korat Š, Bidesi NSR, Bonanno F, et al. Alpha-synuclein PET tracer development-an overview about current efforts. Pharmaceuticals 2021;14(9).

33. Eberling JL, Dave KD, Frasier MA. α-synuclein imaging: a critical need for Parkinson's disease research. J Parkinsons Dis 2013;3(4):565–7.

34. Hsieh C-J, Ferrie JJ, Xu K, et al. Alpha synuclein fibrils contain multiple binding sites for small molecules. ACS Chem Neurosci 2018;9(11):2521–7.

35. Strohäker T, Jung BC, Liou S-H, et al. Structural heterogeneity of α-synuclein fibrils amplified from patient brain extracts. Nat Commun 2019;10(1):5535.

36. Wong DF, Yung B, Dannals RF, et al. In vivo imaging of baboon and human dopamine transporters by positron emission tomography using [11C] WIN 35,428. Synapse 1993;15(2):130–42.

37. Brooks DJ. PET studies on the early and differential diagnosis of Parkinson's disease. Neurology 1993; 43(12 Suppl 6):S6–16.

38. Frey KA, Koeppe RA, Kilbourn MR, et al. Presynaptic monoaminergic vesicles in Parkinson's disease and normal aging. Ann Neurol 1996;40(6):873–84.

39. Cohen AD, Klunk WE. Early detection of Alzheimer's disease using PiB and FDG PET. Neurobiol Dis 2014;117–22, 72 Pt A.

40. Gerhard A, Pavese N, Hotton G, et al. In vivo imaging of microglial activation with [11C](R)-PK11195 PET in idiopathic Parkinson's disease. Neurobiol Dis 2006;21(2):404–12.

41. Maruyama M, Shimada H, Suhara T, et al. Imaging of tau pathology in a tauopathy mouse model and in Alzheimer patients compared to normal controls. Neuron 2013;79(6):1094–108.

42. Foster NL, Heidebrink JL, Clark CM, et al. FDG-PET improves accuracy in distinguishing frontotemporal dementia and Alzheimer's disease. Brain 2007;130(Pt 10):2616–35.

43. Ramlackhansingh AF, Brooks DJ, Greenwood RJ, et al. Inflammation after trauma: microglial activation and traumatic brain injury. Ann Neurol 2011;70(3): 374 83.

44. Walker Z, Moreno E, Thomas A, et al. Clinical usefulness of dopamine transporter SPECT imaging with 123I-FP-CIT in patients with possible dementia with Lewy bodies: randomised study. Br J Psychiatry 2015;206(2):145–52.

45. Sidhu MK, Duncan JS, Sander JW. Neuroimaging in epilepsy. Curr Opin Neurol 2018;31(4):371–8.

46. Chandra PS, Salamon N, Huang J, et al. FDG-PET/MRI coregistration and diffusion-tensor imaging distinguish epileptogenic tubers and cortex in patients with tuberous sclerosis complex: a preliminary report. Epilepsia 2006;47(9):1543–9.

47. Verger A, Kas A, Darcourt J, et al. PET imaging in neuro-oncology: an update and overview of a rapidly growing area. Cancers 2022;14(5):1103.

48. Colavolpe C, Metellus P, Mancini J, et al. Independent prognostic value of pre-treatment 18-FDG-PET in high-grade gliomas. J Neuro Oncol 2011; 107(3):527–35.

49. Ziessman HA, O'Malley JP, Thrall JH. Preface. In: Nuclear medicine. Elsevier; 2006. v-vi.

50. Dunet V, Pomoni A, Hottinger A, et al. Performance of 18F-FET versus 18F-FDG-PET for the diagnosis and grading of brain tumors: systematic review and meta-analysis. Neuro Oncol 2016;18(3): 426–34.

51. Zaragori T, Doyen M, Rech F, et al. Dynamic 18F-FDopa PET imaging for newly-diagnosed gliomas: is a semi-quantitative model sufficient? research square platform LLC. Front Oncol 2021;11: 735257.

52. Sala Q, Metellus P, Taieb D, et al. 18F-DOPA, a clinically available PET tracer to study brain inflammation? Clin Nucl Med 2014;39(4):e283–5.

53. Dutour A, Kumar U, Panetta R, et al. Expression of somatostatin receptor subtypes in human brain tumors. Int J Cancer 1998;76(5):620–7.

54. Rachinger W, Stoecklein VM, Terpolilli NA, et al. Increased 68Ga-DOTATATE uptake in PET imaging discriminates meningioma and tumor-free tissue. J Nucl Med 2015;56(3):347–53.

55. Yang M, Sun J, Bai HX, et al. Diagnostic accuracy of SPECT, PET, and MRS for primary central nervous system lymphoma in HIV patients: a systematic review and meta-analysis. Medicine 2017;96(19): e6676.

56. Tomura N, Kokubun M, Saginoya T, et al. Differentiation between treatment-induced necrosis and recurrent tumors in patients with metastatic brain tumors: comparison among (11)C-Methionine-PET, FDG-PET, MR permeability imaging, and MRI-ADC-preliminary results. AJNR American journal of neuroradiology 2017;38(8):1520–7.

57. Purandare NC, Puranik A, Shah S, et al. Common malignant brain tumors. Nucl Med Commun 2017; 38(12):1109–16.

58. Papin-Michault C, Bonnetaud C, Dufour M, et al. Study of LAT1 expression in brain metastases: towards a better understanding of the results of positron emission tomography using amino acid tracers. PLoS One 2016;11(6):e0157139.

59. Stender J, Kupers R, Rodell A, et al. Quantitative rates of brain glucose metabolism distinguish minimally conscious from vegetative state patients. J Cerebr Blood Flow Metab 2015;35(1):58–65.

60. Sinha P, Conrad GR. Scintigraphy in the confirmation of brain death: Indian context. Indian J Nucl Med 2012;27(1):1–4.

61. Zipursky RB, Meyer JH, Verhoeff NP. PET and SPECT imaging in psychiatric disorders. Can J Psychiatr 2007;52(3):146–57.

62. Miller JM, Hesselgrave N, Ogden RT, et al. Brain serotonin 1A receptor binding as a predictor of treatment outcome in major depressive disorder. Biol Psychiatr 2013;74(10):760–7.

63. Svensson JE, Svanborg C, Plavén-Sigray P, et al. Serotonin transporter availability increases in patients recovering from a depressive episode. Transl Psychiatry 2021;11(1):264.

64. Peciña M, Sikora M, Avery ET, et al. Striatal dopamine D2/3 receptor-mediated neurotransmission in major depression: implications for anhedonia, anxiety and treatment response. Eur Neuropsychopharmacol 2017;27(10):977–86.

65. Holmes SE, Hinz R, Conen S, et al. Elevated translocator protein in anterior cingulate in major depression and a role for inflammation in suicidal thinking: a positron emission tomography study. Biol Psychiatr 2018;83(1):61–9.

66. Mansur RB, Zugman A, Ahmed J, et al. Treatment with a GLP-1R agonist over four weeks promotes weight loss-moderated changes in frontal-striatal brain structures in individuals with mood disorders. Eur Neuropsychopharmacol 2017;27(11): 1153–62.

67. Ota M, Ishikawa M, Sato N, et al. Glutamatergic changes in the cerebral white matter associated with schizophrenic exacerbation. Acta Psychiatr Scand 2012;126(1):72–8.

68. Newberg AB, Moss AS, Monti DA, et al. Positron emission tomography in psychiatric disorders. Ann N Y Acad Sci 2011;1228(1):E13–25.

69. Wong DF, Wagner HN Jr, Tune LE, et al. Positron emission tomography reveals elevated D2 dopamine receptors in drug-naive schizophrenics. Science 1986;234(4783):1558–63.

70. Fusar-Poli P, Meyer-Lindenberg A. Striatal presynaptic dopamine in schizophrenia, part II: meta-analysis of [(18)F/(11)C]-DOPA PET studies. Schizophr Bull 2013;39(1):33–42.

71. Farde L, Sedvall G, Wiesel F-A, et al. Brain dopamine receptors in schizophrenia: PET problems-reply. Arch Gen Psychiatr 1988;45(6):599–600.

72. Egerton A, Brugger S, Raffin M, et al. Anterior cingulate glutamate levels related to clinical status following treatment in first-episode schizophrenia. Neuropsychopharmacology 2012;37(11):2515–21.

73. Kumar JS, Mann JJ. PET tracers for serotonin receptors and their applications. Cent Nerv Syst Agents Med Chem 2014;14(2):96–112.

74. Wang GJ, Volkow ND, Fowler JS, et al. PET studies of the effects of aerobic exercise on human striatal dopamine release. J Nucl Med 2000;41(8):1352–6.

75. Wiers CE, Shumay E, Volkow ND, et al. Effects of depressive symptoms and peripheral DAT methylation on neural reactivity to alcohol cues in alcoholism. Transl Psychiatry 2015;5(9):e648.

76. Kolanko MA, Win Z, Loreto F, et al. Amyloid PET imaging in clinical practice. Practical Neurol 2020; 20(6):451–62.

77. Wong DF, Gjedde A, Wagner HN Jr, et al. Quantification of Neuroreceptors in the living human brain. II. Inhibition studies of receptor density and affinity. J Cerebr Blood Flow Metabol 1986;6(2):147–53.

78. Wong DF, Tauscher J, Gründer G. The role of imaging in proof of concept for CNS drug discovery and development. Neuropsychopharmacology 2009; 34(1):187–203.

79. Catana C. Development of dedicated brain PET imaging devices: recent advances and future perspectives. J Nucl Med : official publication, Society of Nuclear Medicine 2019;60(8):1044–52.

80. Badawi RD, Shi H, Hu P, et al. First human imaging studies with the EXPLORER total-body PET scanner. J Nucl Med : official publication, Society of Nuclear Medicine 2019;60(3):299–303.

81. Sossi V, de Jong HWAM, Barker WC, et al. The second generation HRRT - a multi centre scanner performance investigation. In: IEEE nuclear science symposium conference record. IEEE; 2005.

82. van Velden FHP, Kloet RW, van Berckel DNM, et al. HRRT versus HR+ human brain PET studies: an interscanner test–retest study. J Nucl Med 2009; 50(5):693–702.

83. Conti M, Bendriem B. The new opportunities for high time resolution clinical TOF PET. Clinical and Translational Imaging 2019;7(2):139–47.

84. Carson R, Berg E, Badawi R, et al. Design of the NeuroEXPLORER, a next-generation ultra-high performance human brain PET imager. J Nucl Med 2021;62:1120.

85. Tashima, H., H. Ito, and T. Yamaya. A proposed helmet-PET with a jaw detector enabling high-sensitivity brain imaging. in 2013 IEEE Nuclear Science Symposium and Medical Imaging Conference (2013 NSS/MIC). 2013.

Clinical Applications of Dedicated Breast Positron Emission Tomography

Amy M. Fowler, MD, PhD[a,b,c],*, Kanae K. Miyake, MD, PhD[d],
Yuji Nakamoto, MD, PhD[e]

KEYWORDS

- Dedicated breast PET • Positron emission mammography • Breast-specific positron imaging • FDG
- FES

KEY POINTS

- Breast-specific positron imaging systems provide higher sensitivity than whole-body PET for breast cancer detection.
- Breast-specific positron imaging has similar clinical indications as breast MRI and may be a feasible alternative for patients who have contraindications for breast MRI.
- Further research is needed in developing direct biopsy capability for the prone dedicated breast PET design, methods for reduced radiation dose, and appropriate use criteria.

INTRODUCTION

Nuclear medicine plays an important role for patients with breast cancer. For initial staging of newly diagnosed breast cancer, nuclear medicine examinations are key for determining the number and location of nodal metastases (N stage) and presence or absence of distant metastatic disease (M stage) that will inform prognosis and treatment decisions. Lymphoscintigraphy with ^{99m}Tc-sulfur colloid in conjunction with sentinel lymph node biopsy during initial breast cancer surgery is the gold standard for axillary nodal staging. As bone marrow is a frequent metastatic site for breast cancer, skeletal scintigraphy with ^{99m}Tc-methylene diphosphonate is commonly performed as an adjunct to computed tomography (CT) of the chest, abdomen, and pelvis for initial systemic staging. Whole-body PET/CT with 2-deoxy-2-[^{18}F]fluoro-D-glucose (FDG) is another approach for the initial systemic staging, restaging, and therapy response assessment for patients with breast cancer.[1] PET/CT can also be performed with a newly FDA-approved radiopharmaceutical, 16α-[^{18}F]fluoro-17β-estradiol (FES), for patients with biopsy-proven recurrent or metastatic ER-positive breast cancer to guide treatment decisions.[2]

Although useful for extra-axillary nodal and distant metastatic disease assessment, whole-body FDG PET/CT is not recommended for primary breast cancer detection, for characterization of breast masses as benign or malignant, or for determining the size and extent of disease localized within the breast (T stage) due to limited spatial resolution for sub-centimeter cancers.[3,4] This technical constraint of whole-body scanners fueled the development of dedicated breast imaging devices with detectors placed closer to the breast for improved spatial resolution.[5] Several review articles have been published detailing the research in this area.[6–11] This review provides an update on the clinical applications of dedicated breast PET.

[a] Department of Radiology, University of Wisconsin School of Medicine and Public Health, 600 Highland Avenue, Madison, WI 53792-3252, USA; [b] Department of Medical Physics, University of Wisconsin-Madison; [c] University of Wisconsin Carbone Cancer Center, Madison, WI, USA; [d] Department of Advanced Medical Imaging Research, Graduate School of Medicine Kyoto University, Kyoto, Japan; [e] Department of Diagnostic Imaging and Nuclear Medicine, Graduate School of Medicine Kyoto University, Kyoto, Japan
* Corresponding author. University of Wisconsin School of Medicine and Public Health, 600 Highland Avenue, Madison, WI 53792-3252.
E-mail address: afowler@uwhealth.org

PET Clin 19 (2024) 105–117
https://doi.org/10.1016/j.cpet.2023.06.004
1556-8598/24/© 2023 Elsevier Inc. All rights reserved.

IMAGE ACQUISITION AND INTERPRETATION

Another article in this journal issue focuses on the recent advances in breast PET instrumentation.[12] To summarize here briefly, breast-specific positron imaging systems use 2 types of configurations. The planar or "opposite-type" design consists of 2 opposing parallel planar detectors called positron emission mammography (PEM). For PEM, the breast is stabilized using mild compression with images acquired in the same views as conventional x-ray mammography with the patient seated. The other configuration uses a ring-shaped detector and acquires images with the patient in the prone position, similar to breast MRI. This "ring-shaped" design, termed dedicated breast PET (dbPET), provides full 3-dimensional images. Other organ-targeted PET imaging devices can be used for imaging the brain, extremities, or heart, as well as for breast imaging.[13] Several dbPET devices that are coupled with other modalities such as x-ray mammography,[14] digital breast tomosynthesis,[15] CT,[16] and diffuse optical tomography[17] are being developed. The in-plane spatial resolution of breast-specific positron imaging systems is typically 1 to 2 mm compared with 4 to 6 mm with whole-body PET scanners, which enables smaller lesion detection.[18–21]

Updated clinical practice guidelines for the performance of high-resolution breast PET have been published.[22] As with whole-body FDG PET/CT, patients are instructed to fast for at least 4 to 6 hours. The intravenously injected activity of FDG is typically the same as for whole-body PET/CT (3.0–3.7 MBq/kg body weight). Published reports have ranged from 90 to 370 MBq and there are ongoing research efforts to reduce the dose, as described later. Image acquisition typically begins 60 minutes after FDG injection or 90 minutes postinjection if dbPET is performed after whole-body PET. For PEM, craniocaudal and mediolateral oblique views of each breast are acquired for 10 minutes per view (40-minute total scan time). For dbPET, images are acquired for 5 to 15 minutes per breast.

A key aspect of breast imaging is the use of standardized reporting for mammography, ultrasound, and breast MRI with final assessment categories linked with specific management recommendations used in clinical practice. This approach provides a common language for communicating with other radiologists, breast center nurses, referring physicians, and patients for optimal patient care. It also provides a method for standardized data collection and comparison of results of research studies across multiple institutions. For breast-specific positron imaging, standardized terminology has also been developed to describe and interpret findings in a consistent and reproducible manner.[23,24] Based on morphology and distribution descriptors, mass uptake and segmental and focal distributions of nonmass uptake have the highest likelihood of malignancy.[25–27] The lexicon uses similar terminology as the American College of Radiology Breast Imaging Reporting and Data System for breast MRI[28] but also contains some unique descriptors. Experienced breast imaging radiologists who completed a 2-hour training module in PEM interpretation for a multi-institutional clinical trial in the Unites States achieved high diagnostic accuracy and interobserver agreement.[29] Finally, breast-specific positron imaging examinations should be interpreted in the context of all other breast imaging results available, together with clinical history about previous breast biopsies and treatment.

BIOPSY CAPABILITY

Because certain lesions may only be visualized on PET, an essential feature of breast-specific positron imaging systems is to provide biopsy capability. These are typically developed as add-on options compatible with existing scanners. A PEM-guided biopsy system is commercially available that uses a stereotactic method for lesion targeting.[30–32] A prospective, multicenter study of 19 patients demonstrated that all 24 suspicious breast lesions were successfully targeted and sampled using PEM-guided biopsy.[31] Additionally, a small, single-center prospective study of 20 patients demonstrated feasibility of performing diagnostic PEM imaging and PEM-guided biopsy on the same day, which decreases radiation dose to the patient and staff as well as eliminating an additional patient visit before surgery.[32] Compared with MRI-guided biopsy, specimen imaging can be performed for PEM-guided biopsy to confirm FDG activity within the biopsy cores indicating adequate sampling.[31–33] A recent investigation has also reported integrating ultrasound-guided core needle biopsy with PEM localization as an alternative approach to direct PEM-guided biopsy.[34] Biopsy systems for dbPET systems remain in technical development and are not yet available for clinical use.[35]

DIAGNOSTIC PERFORMANCE

Several studies have evaluated the diagnostic performance of breast-specific positron imaging systems for cancer detection. A meta-analysis of 8 studies including 873 women with known or suspected breast cancer imaged with PEM reported

85% pooled sensitivity, 79% pooled specificity, and an area under the receiver operating characteristic curve (AUC) of 0.88 overall.[36] The pooled sensitivity was 86% for invasive breast cancer and 81% for in situ disease.[36] In 2020, a subsequent meta-analysis of 5 studies including 722 women with breast cancer demonstrated better sensitivity, negative predictive value, and accuracy of PEM compared with whole-body PET for primary breast cancer detection.[37] Specificity and positive predictive value was similar between the 2 modalities. For dbPET, recent large studies involving up to 938 women also found increased sensitivity for breast cancer detection compared with whole-body PET/CT, particularly for T1 stage (<2 cm) and subcentimeter tumors, lower grade tumors, and ductal carcinoma in situ (DCIS).[38,39] Other prospective studies of the diagnostic performance of dbPET systems have been published.[40–43]

A recent prospective study by Hashimoto and colleagues aimed to determine the sensitivity of dbPET in patients with newly diagnosed breast cancer and compare with the sensitivity of mammography, ultrasound, breast MRI, and whole-body PET/MRI.[41] The study included 82 women with 84 malignant tumors (11 DCIS and 73 invasive carcinoma). For all tumors, the sensitivity was 81.2% for mammography, 98.8% for ultrasound, 98.6% for breast MRI, 86.9% for whole-body PET/MRI, and 89.2% for dbPET. For the 11 cases of DCIS and 22 small invasive cancers (≤2 cm), the sensitivity of dbPET (84.9%) tended to be higher than that of whole-body PET/MRI (69.7%), although not statistically significant (P = .095). Of note, the 7 cancers detected only by dbPET but not with whole-body PET/MRI were 4 cases of DCIS and 3 small cases of invasive ductal carcinoma (3–9 mm maximal diameter).

A large retrospective study by Sasada and colleagues aimed to evaluate the sensitivity of dbPET to detect the various histologic types of breast cancer.[39] The study included 938 patients with 1021 lesions and found the sensitivity of dbPET was 90.3%, compared with 75.6% with whole-body PET/CT, across all tumor types.[39] For subcentimeter tumors, the sensitivity of dbPET (81.9%) was higher than that of whole-body PET/CT (52.4%).[39] The only subtypes for which dbPET had low sensitivity was tubular carcinoma (61.5%) and lobular carcinoma in situ (27.3%), which is treated as a high-risk lesion.[39] For the 158 cases of DCIS, the sensitivity of dbPET was 82.3%, which was higher than that of whole-body PET/CT (50.0%).[39] Other studies have reported the sensitivity of PEM or dbPET to detect DCIS as 41%,[44] 80%,[45] 81.8%,[41] 90%,[46] 90.9%,[47] and

91%.[48] Thus, breast-specific positron imaging has high sensitivity to detect most histologic subtypes of breast cancer including DCIS.

CLINICAL APPLICATIONS

Breast-specific positron imaging has similar clinical applications as breast MRI and may be a reasonable alternative for patients who are not candidates for breast MRI (claustrophobia, gadolinium-based contrast agent allergy, cardiac pacemaker, and severe renal impairment).[22,44,46] The clinical scenarios for which breast-specific positron imaging has been investigated include local tumor staging for patients with newly diagnosed breast cancer for surgical planning, neoadjuvant therapy response assessment, tumor phenotyping, problem solving for indeterminate conventional imaging results, and screening. Another potential clinical application is detecting local disease recurrence within the breast in patients with a personal history of treated breast cancer. Appropriate Use Criteria has not yet been developed by the Society of Nuclear Medicine and Molecular Imaging.

Local Staging for Newly Diagnosed Breast Cancer

Accurate local tumor staging is important for determining clinical T stage for prognosis as well as for surgical planning to decide between breast conserving surgery or mastectomy. Breast-specific positron imaging may reveal occult malignancy not identified on mammography and ultrasound. Detection of multicentric disease in the ipsilateral breast or detection of malignancy in the contralateral breast can lead to a critical change in clinical management.[49,50] Case examples of dbPET performed for patients with newly diagnosed breast cancer are shown in **Figs. 1** and **2**.

Breast MRI can be used in addition to mammography and ultrasound for local preoperative staging and screening the contralateral breast due to its higher sensitivity, although this is not universal. There have been 2 large prospective studies comparing PEM with breast MRI for preoperative local tumor staging involving 388 and 208 newly diagnosed patients with breast cancer, respectively.[44,46] Both studies showed that the sensitivity of PEM was comparable to breast MRI for detecting additional unsuspected cancers in the ipsilateral breast.[44,46] The specificity of PEM was comparable[46] or better[44] than breast MRI. In the study by Berg and colleagues, the sensitivity for detecting additional foci of DCIS was relatively low for both breast MRI (39%) and PEM (41%).[44] However, sensitivity for DCIS was improved

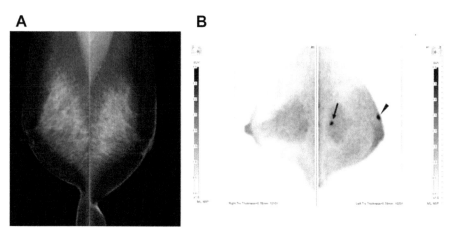

Fig. 1. A postmenopausal woman in her 50s with eczema-like changes around the left nipple, which was diagnosed as Paget disease by biopsy. To evaluate for an associated malignancy within the breast, mammography (*A* [MLO view]) and ultrasound were performed but showed no suspicious findings. FDG dbPET demonstrated an intense focus in the central left breast (*B* [ML view], *arrow*), which was proven as DCIS by subsequent partial mastectomy. An arrowhead (*B*) on the skin above the areola indicates inflammatory change after biopsy. Diffuse skin uptake of the left breast was thought primarily due to the reaction from skin phototherapy pursued at the patient's own discretion before the diagnosis of breast cancer.

(57%) when PEM was added to breast MRI.[44] In the study by Schilling and colleagues, there was no statistically significant difference between the sensitivity of PEM (90%) and breast MRI (83%) to detect the 30 index lesions that were DCIS.[46] No studies have been published yet comparing dbPET with breast MRI for preoperative local staging.

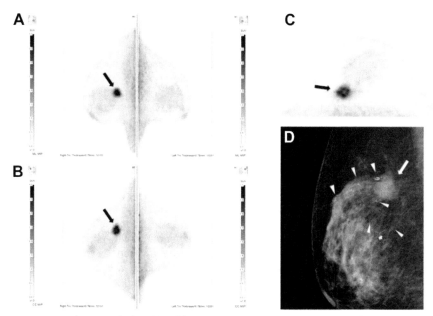

Fig. 2. A postmenopausal woman in her 60s with HR-positive/HER2-positive invasive breast carcinoma (no special type) in the right breast. FDG dbPET was performed instead of MRI for surgical planning because she had a pacemaker. DbPET showed intense irregular mass uptake with rim pattern (*A–C, arrows*), corresponding to the pathologically proven invasive cancer. Rim uptake can be one of typical findings indicative of invasive cancer. There was no additional uptake on dbPET; however, a few centimeters of DCIS was present around the invasive carcinoma (*arrow*) on surgical pathology, as indicated on digital mammography as suspicious microcalcifications (*D, arrowheads*). This case illustrates both advantages of dbPET (availability for patients with contraindications for breast MRI, good sensitivity for invasive cancers, and the ability to depict uptake morphology, which supports the diagnosis) and disadvantages (reduced sensitivity for DCIS).

A few studies have investigated the frequency of additional incidental abnormal FDG uptake detected with dbPET and percentage of malignancy in patients with breast cancer. A retrospective study by Satoh and colleagues included a total of 627 women who underwent dbPET, which included 44 women with breast cancer undergoing pretherapy imaging, 98 posttherapy, and 15 women suspected of breast cancer based on mammography, ultrasound, palpation, or blood test abnormalities.[25] For each subset population, the new cancer detection rates were 4.5% (2/44), 2.0% (2/98), and 13.3% (2/15), respectively.[25] The positive predictive values were 50.0% (2/4), 42.9% (3/7), 66.7% (2/3), respectively.[25] In a retrospective study by Sasada and colleagues involving 709 patients with breast cancer, the incidental cancer detection rate was 10.5% (20/190).[26] A subsequent study by this research group involving 1076 patients with breast cancer found a similar incidental cancer detection rate of 11.6% (32/276).[27] Thus, the frequency of incidental findings detected with dbPET ranges from 7.6% to 20.9%, with 4.5% to 11.6% of these incidental findings being malignant in patients with known breast cancer.

Neoadjuvant Therapy Response Assessment

Neoadjuvant therapy is a commonly used approach for breast cancer management. A complete pathologic response after neoadjuvant therapy may allow less-extensive breast and axillary surgery and also inform patient prognosis. Imaging can be used to identify nonresponders early to enable a change in therapy and for final surgical planning based on residual disease at the completion of neoadjuvant therapy. The American College of Radiology Appropriate Use Criteria for monitoring response to neoadjuvant therapy for breast cancer includes ultrasound, digital breast tomosynthesis, and breast MRI.[51] A case example of dbPET and breast MRI performed before and after neoadjuvant chemotherapy is shown in **Fig. 3**.

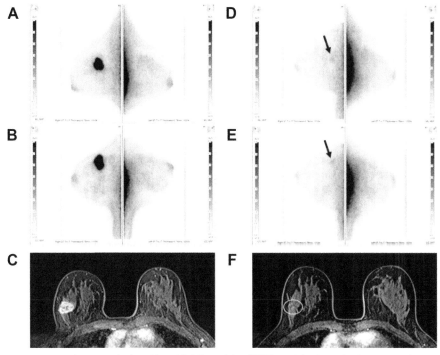

Fig. 3. A postmenopausal woman in her 40s with HR-positive/HER2-positive invasive breast carcinoma (no special type) in the right breast. Before neoadjuvant treatment with chemotherapy and HER2-targeted therapy, FDG dbPET showed intense mass uptake in the upper outer right breast (A, B), and dynamic contrast-enhanced breast MRI showed mass enhancement (C), corresponding to the tumor. After neoadjuvant therapy completion, dbPET (D, E, arrows) demonstrated remarkable decrease of the tumor uptake but residual faint mass uptake was seen. Posttherapy MRI showed subtle enhancement consisting of clustered 3 foci (nonmass enhancement) (F, circle). Thus, it was suspected that small residual invasive cancers or residual DCIS remained. On surgical pathology, 1.1 cm of residual invasive carcinoma within prominent fibrotic change of the tumor bed was identified. Combination use of dbPET and MRI may be helpful to increase confidence in the diagnosis of residual tumor after neoadjuvant therapy for surgical planning and prognosis.

There have been a few studies investigating the performance of breast-specific positron imaging for the assessment of neoadjuvant therapy response. As an early biomarker of therapy response, a decrease in FDG uptake on PEM after the first cycle of neoadjuvant chemotherapy has been shown to correlate with final pathologic response across all molecular subtypes.[52] Similarly, the ability to measure early neoadjuvant chemotherapy response with dbPET that precedes anatomic changes on breast MRI was highlighted in a case report by Jones and colleagues in a multicenter adaptive neoadjuvant therapy clinical trial (I-SPY 2).[53]

For detection of residual disease after completion of neoadjuvant chemotherapy, PEM and dbPET have been shown to be more sensitive and more accurate than whole-body PET/CT.[54–56] The prospective study by Tokuda and colleagues compared the performance of dbPET, whole-body PET/CT, and breast MRI for determining pathologic complete response after neoadjuvant chemotherapy for 29 women with breast cancer.[57] The study found that dbPET is a better predictor of pathologic complete response after completion of neoadjuvant chemotherapy than whole-body PET/CT. Furthermore, a reduction in standardized uptake values corrected for lean body mass (SUL_{peak}) greater than 82% was an independent predictor of pathologic complete response in multivariate analysis.

Tumor Phenotyping

Breast cancer is a heterogenous disease with multiple molecular subtypes and various clinical outcomes. Several studies have examined the association between imaging features obtained with FDG dbPET and clinicopathological features of breast cancer. As seen with whole-body PET/CT, SUV_{max} of dbPET is higher with clinical T stages 2 to 4, nuclear grades 2 to 3, Ki67 proliferation index 20% or greater, ER-negative, human epidermal growth factor receptor 2 (HER2)-positive, and lymph node-positive breast cancer.[41,58] When matched for SUV_{max}, a heterogeneous intratumoral distribution of FDG uptake was associated with high nuclear grade and high Ki67 proliferation.[58] Similarly, a rim uptake pattern on dbPET was associated with aggressive pathologic features including high nuclear grade, high Ki67 proliferation, and triple-negative subtypes[59] and was seen more often on dbPET than whole-body PET/CT.[59] Tumor areas without FDG uptake correlated with central necrosis or fibrosis on hematoxylin and eosin staining.[58,59] It is important to note that tumor phenotype information provided by

dbPET remains insufficient to consider clinical use as a reliable surrogate measure for pathologic assessment.

Breast-specific positron imaging may also provide information regarding the tumor microenvironment. FDG uptake in breast cancer reflects uptake by tumor cells as well as by the associated tumor microenvironment including immune cells. Tumor infiltrating lymphocytes (TILs) are abundant in triple-negative and HER2-positive breast cancers and are a predictor of pathologic response to neoadjuvant chemotherapy. The study by Sasada and colleagues demonstrated a correlation between high TILs and high SUV_{max} using dbPET but not with whole-body PET/CT for 125 invasive breast cancers.[60]

DbPET has also been investigated as a method to differentiate between indolent and aggressive DCIS to reduce overdiagnosis, a frequently cited drawback of screening mammography. The study by Grana-Lopez and colleagues included 139 cases of pure DCIS confirmed at surgery (50 high risk and 89 low risk).[61] The sensitivity and specificity of dbPET to distinguish between indolent and potentially aggressive DCIS was 90% and 92%, respectively.[61] Accurate identification of indolent DCIS noninvasively with dbPET could support active surveillance rather than surgical excision for clinical management.

Problem Solving

One clinical application of interest for all types of functional imaging, including breast-specific positron imaging, is to avoid unnecessary biopsies prompted by false-positive findings on conventional breast imaging (mammography, ultrasound, MRI). A prospective single-center study by Grana-Lopez and colleagues included 50 women with 60 Breast Imaging Reporting and Data System (BI-RADS) category 4 (suspicious) breast lesions who underwent breast MRI and dbPET before biopsy for histologic confirmation.[62] The study found that the sensitivity and specificity of dbPET was 50% and 76%, respectively.[62] The false-negative lesions that resulted in low sensitivity included 2 invasive ductal carcinomas located in the posterior breast outside of the field-of-view, a 10-mm size invasive lobular carcinoma, and 5 cases of DCIS.[62] The authors concluded that dbPET should not be recommended to resolve suspicious mammographic or sonographic findings given the relatively high rate of false-negative results.

The study by Bitencourt and colleagues aimed to determine the diagnostic accuracy of PEM to identify breast cancer in patients with suspicious calcifications on mammography.[63] This prospective, single-center study involved 40 patients.[63] PEM detected all cases of invasive carcinoma and high-grade DCIS with one false-positive result (fibroadenoma) and one false-negative result (intermediate-grade DCIS).[63] The authors concluded that PEM may be helpful in distinguishing benign from malignant calcifications on mammography.[63]

A drawback of breast MRI is its moderate specificity and possibility to yield false-positive findings. A pilot study by Malhotra and colleagues investigated the utility of dbPET in 10 patients with breast cancer and indeterminate lesions on preoperative breast MRI.[64] The study concluded that dbPET was not able to reliably characterize MRI-indeterminate lesions as benign or malignant in the small patient cohort.[64] Thus, based on these limited studies, breast-specific positron imaging should not be used to avoid further workup and biopsy of suspicious findings on mammography, ultrasound, and breast MRI.

Supplemental Screening

Supplemental screening for women with mammographically dense breasts or those with elevated lifetime risk of breast cancer include ultrasound, breast MRI, and molecular breast imaging with ^{99m}Tc-sestamibi. The American College of Radiology Appropriateness Criteria for supplemental breast cancer screening based on breast density states that there is limited literature regarding the use of breast-specific positron imaging for supplemental screening.[65] One study reported a 2.3% (6/265) cancer detection rate using PEM in 265 women (165 without breast symptoms) participating in an FDG PET cancer-screening program in Japan.[66] In the study by Satoh and colleagues, the cancer detection rate of dbPET in the subset population of 423 women undergoing cancer screening was 1.7% (7/423) with a positive predictive value of 26.9% (7/26).[25] However, these early studies are small in size and included a mixed population of women with and without breast symptoms, which may have resulted in such high cancer detection rates and positive predictive value. Future studies are needed to determine the diagnostic performance in typical screening settings for asymptomatic women.

RADIATION DOSE CONSIDERATIONS

A barrier to the use of breast-specific positron imaging for supplemental breast cancer screening is the current radiation exposure associated with the examination (3.5 mSv effective dose equivalent from 185 MBq FDG).[22] Although this amount is comparable to natural background radiation and considered negligible risk, it is more than the

amount from digital mammography (0.5 mSv) or from molecular breast imaging (2.5 mSv from 300 MBq ^{99m}Tc-sestamibi). Furthermore, supplemental screening with ultrasound and breast MRI has no associated radiation exposure.

Ongoing research efforts have focused on methods to reduce the radiation dose, which would address a major barrier to the clinical utilization of breast-specific positron imaging. The possibility of obtaining clinically acceptable image quality with lower injected tracer activity was supported by a case report of a patient with invasive ductal carcinoma, which was adequately imaged with PEM using a much lower amount of FDG (estimated 25.9 MBq) than the standard 185 to 370 MBq activity.[33] Using phantom experiments, MacDonald and colleagues demonstrated that the detection sensitivity of PEM remained above 90% for injected ^{18}F activities as low as 100 MBq for lesion at least 8 mm in diameter.[67] However, in a subsequent study with 30 patients with breast cancer imaged with PEM at 60 and 120 minutes postinjection using standard injected activity and one-half activity, these investigators found trends of lower lesion detection sensitivity with lower image counts that persisted despite a longer uptake time.[68] The authors concluded that to obtain the highest interpretation accuracy the standard injected activity should not be lowered.

Additional research with dbPET systems has further explored dose-reduction techniques. The ring-type design of dbPET with detectors completely surrounding the breast allows for increased photon detection and fully 3-dimensional, isotropic tomographic imaging, which may be better suited for low-dose imaging than the planar-type design with anisotropic spatial resolution. Using simulated dose-reduced images of 28 patients with abnormal FDG uptake on dbPET, Satoh and colleagues demonstrated clinically acceptable image quality using 25% injected FDG activity, which corresponds to a radiation dose of 0.9 mSv (roughly twice that of digital mammography).[69] A subsequent study by this research group that imaged 9 women with dbPET at 60 minutes and 90 minutes after 50% injected FDG activity demonstrated sufficient image quality for clinical use.[70] Artificial intelligence and deep learning models are promising techniques to improve the quality of low count dbPET images and facilitate further dose reduction for breast-specific positron imaging.[71]

ADDITIONAL CONSIDERATIONS

There are other technical, biological, and practical challenges with breast-specific positron imaging.

These devices have inherently limited evaluation of the axilla and difficulty visualizing far posterior lesions near the chest wall, particularly with the prone design.[41–45,47,62,72–74] However, modifications to the imaging table have been shown to increase the amount of breast tissue in the field-of-view.[41,74] As an alternative approach to increase the field-of-view, a dedicated total breast PET system has been designed using a novel "stadium" shaped ring geometry to simultaneously image both breasts, axilla, and mediastinum with improved breast lesion detectability compared with whole-body PET in a simulation study.[75] Another ring-type dbPET system (named BRPET) has also been designed with the goal of improved visualization of posterior breast tissue using vertically slanted light guides to partially extend the scintillation crystal array into the table aperture.[76]

Furthermore, some tumor types may not have sufficient levels of glucose metabolism to be detected using FDG despite the higher spatial resolution of breast-specific positron imaging. These are potential causes for false-negative examinations. The study by Sasada and colleagues in 2018 with 265 patients found that 7 of the 24 cancers that were not detected by dbPET were low-grade tumors.[47] A larger subsequent study by this group of 938 patients with breast cancer observed a relatively low sensitivity of dbPET for detecting tubular carcinoma (61.5%), a well-differentiated, indolent type of breast cancer.[39] In the study by Hashimoto and colleagues of 82 patients with breast cancer, 2 cases of invasive lobular carcinoma and a case of mucinous carcinoma were not detected by dbPET.[41]

Although breast-specific positron imaging has moderately high specificity, efforts to further reduce false-positive examinations are important. FDG uptake is not specific to cancers but various benign lesions can also accumulate FDG, such as intraductal papillomas, complicated cysts, fibroadenomas, and inflammation.[26] Breast-specific positron imaging has a greater chance of detecting benign uptake due to its increased sensitivity for subtle uptake. Dual-time-point imaging has been shown to improve sensitivity and specificity for distinguishing benign from malignant breast lesions using whole body FDG PET,[77,78] and may likely have a beneficial effect for dbPET imaging. In addition, the detector geometry of dbPET is often associated with nonpathological dot-like uptake, called *noise*, which can be especially problematic when performing breast-specific PET aimed to the detection of small breast cancers, that is, screening, and should be considered when using pixel-based uptake values (SUV_{max}) that are susceptible to statistical noise. It has been reported that the image quality especially around the detector edge tends to be decreased[79] and that intense radioactivity outside of the field-of-view near the chest wall, that is, FDG activity in the myocardium, is associated with increased noise.[80] A recent study demonstrated that reproducibility assessment using 2 sets of reconstructed dbPET images may be helpful to differentiate true pathologic uptake from noise.[81] Technical efforts, such as the development of artificial intelligence-based image reconstruction, have been made to improve image quality with less noise.[71] Such technologies are also expected to allow shorter image acquisition time with acceptable image quality, thereby reducing the physical burden on patients.

Practical challenges with breast-specific positron imaging include availability, insurance coverage, and lack of information on its cost effectiveness. In the United States, there is limited clinical implementation with many private insurers categorizing this technology as investigational citing insufficient data on clinical impact. However in Japan, breast PET has been covered by insurance when it is performed with conventional whole-body PET/CT since 2013.[22]

FUTURE RESEARCH
Radiomics and Machine Learning

Radiomics is an emerging approach for extracting large amounts of image features that can uncover tumor characteristics not appreciated by visual assessment. A few studies have used radiomics and texture analysis of dbPET images to explore associations between imaging features and tumor biologic characteristics such as T category, N category, Ki67 proliferation, and molecular subtype. In a study of 127 patients, Morosco and colleagues found that 9 out of 10 features extracted from dbPET images revealed new and stronger correlations with immunohistochemical subtypes compared with previous studies with whole-body PET/CT.[82] In a pilot study of 10 women locally advanced breast cancer, Hathi and colleagues also demonstrated statistically significant differences in spatial heterogeneity features between dbPET and whole-body PET/CT, which the authors suggest are mainly driven by the higher sensitivity of dbPET.[83] However, using a different ring-type dbPET system, the study published by Satoh and colleagues involving 44 women with breast cancer found equivalent predictive ability of tumor characteristics using texture analysis with whole-body PET/CT and dbPET.[84]

Machine learning algorithms have also been used with dbPET for distinguishing benign from malignant breast lesions and for predicting axillary lymph node status. In a study of 105 women, Satoh and colleagues evaluated the diagnostic accuracy of a support vector model for breast lesions smaller than 2 cm with abnormal FDG uptake on dbPET.[85] The model, which included age, maximum standardized uptake value, total lesion glycolysis, and lesion-to-contralateral background ratio, had high diagnostic accuracy (AUC = 0.86) for distinguishing breast cancer from benign lesions, and thus may be a supporting tool for diagnosis of small breast cancers. In a study of 290 women with early-stage breast cancer, Cheng and colleagues developed a machine learning integrated model using dbPET radiomics features and clinicopathologic characteristics for predicting axillary nodal staging.[86] The negative predictive value was 97% in the clinical N0 subgroup with 93% positive predictive value for the clinical N1 subgroup.[86]

Radiopharmaceuticals Beyond 2-deoxy-2-[18F]fluoro-ᴅ-glucose

Potential applications of breast-specific positron imaging may also evolve as new radiopharmaceuticals continue to grow beyond FDG. FES is a radiolabeled estrogen compound that binds to estrogen receptor, a key tumor biomarker for selecting endocrine therapy. A feasibility study by Jones and colleagues involved 6 patients with ER-positive breast cancer imaged with FES dbPET, which showed potential clinical utility as a noninvasive approach to characterize primary ER-positive breast cancer for guiding treatment selection and measuring therapy response.[87]

^{64}Cu-TP3805 is a PET imaging agent with high affinity for vasoactive intestinal and pituitary adenylate cyclase activating peptide 1 (VPAC1) receptors, a G-protein coupled receptor expressed in breast cancer.[88] A feasibility study of 19 women with biopsy-proven breast cancer underwent PEM imaging with ^{64}Cu-TP3805 with promising results, as all lesions were detected by ^{64}Cu-TP3805, with rapid uptake within 15 minutes after injection.[88] The authors proposed further investigation into the use of ^{64}Cu-TP3805 PEM for distinguishing malignant from benign breast lesions and for exploring the development of ^{67}Cu-TP3805 as a targeted radiotherapy agent.

Several other PET radiopharmaceuticals have been investigated for breast cancer imaging using whole-body PET/CT or PET/MRI. These include ^{18}F-fluorofuranylnorprogesterone for progesterone receptor,[89,90] ^{89}Zr-trastuzumab for HER2,[91] ^{18}F-fluoromisonidazole for hypoxia,[92] and ^{18}F-fluorothymidine for proliferation.[93] Imaging fibroblast-activation protein in invasive breast cancer with simultaneous PET/MRI has demonstrated strong uptake of ^{68}Ga-FAPI-46 in primary breast tumors and lymph node metastases.[94] Future studies combining these targeted tracers with dbPET devices may reveal important information regarding local tumor heterogeneity and neoadjuvant therapy response.

SUMMARY

Designed for increased spatial resolution, breast-specific positron imaging systems provide higher sensitivity than whole-body PET for breast cancer detection. Although breast-specific positron imaging systems are not widely used in clinical practice in the United States, there are increasing clinical data published by several international sites, mainly Japan. Further research is necessary into the appropriate clinical applications for breast-specific positron imaging to provide clinically significant information to guide management and treatment decisions for patients with breast cancer. Continued technical innovation using radiomics and deep learning techniques, as well as the exploration of radiopharmaceuticals beyond FDG, will likely contribute to the evolving future clinical applications for breast-specific positron imaging.

DISCLOSURE SUMMARY

A.M. Fowler receives book chapter royalty from Elsevier, Inc and has served on an advisory board for GE Healthcare, United States. The Department of Radiology at the University of Wisconsin School of Medicine and Public Health receives research support from GE Healthcare. The Department of Diagnostic Imaging and Nuclear Medicine, Graduate School of Medicine Kyoto University received research support from Shimadzu Cooperation and Midtown Clinic.

CLINICS CARE POINTS

- Updated clinical practice guidelines for the performance of high-resolution breast PET have been published. The clinical applications for breast-specific positron imaging are similar to breast MRI including preoperative local staging and neoadjuvant therapy response assessment.

- Breast-specific positron imaging exams should be interpreted in the context of all other breast imaging results available, together with clinical history about previous breast biopsies and treatment.

- A standardized lexicon should be used to describe and interpret findings in a consistent and reproducible manner. Based on current evidence, breast-specific positron imaging should not be used to avoid further work-up and biopsy of suspicious findings on mammography, ultrasound, and breast MRI.

ACKNOWLEDGMENTS

The authors acknowledge the University of Wisconsin Carbone Cancer Center Support Grant P30 CA014520, the Department of Radiology, University of Wisconsin School of Medicine and Public Health, and the Department of Breast Surgery and the Department of Diagnostic Imaging and Nuclear Medicine, Graduate School of Medicine Kyoto University.

REFERENCES

1. Fowler AM, Cho SY. PET imaging for breast cancer. Radiol Clin North Am 2021;59(5):725–35.
2. Ulaner GA, Mankoff DA, Clark AS, et al. Summary: appropriate Use criteria for estrogen receptor-targeted PET imaging with 16α-(18)F-Fluoro-17β-Fluoroestradiol. J Nucl Med 2023;64(3):351–4.
3. Kumar R, Chauhan A, Zhuang H, et al. Clinicopathologic factors associated with false negative FDG-PET in primary breast cancer. Breast Cancer Res Treat 2006;98(3):267–74.
4. Avril N, Rose CA, Schelling M, et al. Breast imaging with positron emission tomography and fluorine-18 fluorodeoxyglucose: use and limitations. J Clin Oncol 2000;18(20):3495–502.
5. Thompson CJ, Murthy K, Weinberg IN, et al. Feasibility study for positron emission mammography. Med Phys 1994;21(4):529–38.
6. Narayanan D, Berg WA. Dedicated breast gamma camera imaging and breast PET: current status and future directions. Pet Clin 2018;13(3):363–81.
7. Collarino A, Fuoco V, Pereira Arias-Bouda LM, et al. Novel frontiers of dedicated molecular imaging in breast cancer diagnosis. Transl Cancer Res 2017;S295–306.
8. Miyake KK, Nakamoto Y, Togashi K. Current status of dedicated breast PET imaging. Curr Radiol Rep 2016;4(4):16.
9. Hruska CB, O'Connor MK. Nuclear imaging of the breast: translating achievements in instrumentation into clinical use. Med Phys 2013;40(5):050901.
10. Surti S. Radionuclide methods and instrumentation for breast cancer detection and diagnosis. Semin Nucl Med 2013;43(4):271–80.
11. Hsu DF, Freese DL, Levin CS. Breast-dedicated radionuclide imaging systems. J Nucl Med 2016; 57(Suppl 1):40s–5s.
12. Surti S. Advances in breast PET instrumentation. PET Clin. in pres.
13. Stiles J, Baldassi B, Bubon O, et al. Evaluation of a high-sensitivity organ-targeted PET camera. Sensors 2022;22(13):4678.
14. Zeng C, Kinahan PE, Qian H, et al. Simulation study of quantitative precision of the PET/X dedicated breast PET scanner. J Med Imaging 2017;4(4):045502.
15. Krishnamoorthy S, Vent T, Barufaldi B, et al. Evaluating attenuation correction strategies in a dedicated, single-gantry breast PET-tomosynthesis scanner. Phys Med Biol 2020;65(23):235028.
16. Raylman RR, Van Kampen W, Stolin AV, et al. A dedicated breast-PET/CT scanner: evaluation of basic performance characteristics. Med Phys 2018;45(4):1603–13.
17. Shi Y, Wang Y, Zhou J, et al. DH-Mammo PET: a dual-head positron emission mammography system for breast imaging. Phys Med Biol 2022;67(20).
18. Moliner L, Gonzalez AJ, Soriano A, et al. Design and evaluation of the MAMMI dedicated breast PET. Med Phys 2012;39(9):5393–404.
19. Luo WD, Anashkin E, Matthews CG. Performance evaluation of a PEM scanner using the NEMA NU 4-2008 small animal PET standards. IEEE Trans Nucl Sci 2010;57(1):94–103.
20. Raylman RR, Majewski S, Smith MF, et al. The positron emission mammography/tomography breast imaging and biopsy system (PEM/PET): design, construction and phantom-based measurements. Phys Med Biol 2008;53(3):637–53.
21. Miyake KK, Matsumoto K, Inoue M, et al. Performance evaluation of a new dedicated breast PET scanner using NEMA NU4-2008 standards. J Nucl Med 2014;55(7):1198–203.
22. Satoh Y, Kawamoto M, Kubota K, et al. Clinical practice guidelines for high-resolution breast PET, 2019 edition. Ann Nucl Med 2021;35(3):406–14.
23. Narayanan D, Madsen KS, Kalinyak JE, et al. Interpretation of positron emission mammography: feature analysis and rates of malignancy. AJR Am J Roentgenol 2011;196(4):956–70.
24. Miyake KK, Kataoka M, Ishimori T, et al. A proposed dedicated breast PET lexicon: standardization of description and reporting of radiotracer uptake in the breast. Diagnostics 2021;11(7):1267.
25. Satoh Y, Motosugi U, Omiya Y, et al. Unexpected abnormal uptake in the breasts at dedicated breast PET: Incidentally detected small cancers or Nonmalignant features? AJR Am J Roentgenol 2019;212(2):443–9.
26. Sasada S, Masumoto N, Kimura Y, et al. Classification of abnormal findings on ring-type dedicated breast PET for the detection of breast cancer. Anticancer Res 2020;40(6):3491–7.
27. Sasada S, Masumoto N, Emi A, et al. Malignant prediction of incidental findings using ring-type dedicated breast positron emission tomography. Sci Rep 2022;12(1):1144.

28. Morris EA, Comstock C, Lee C, et al. ACR BI-RADS Magnetic Resonance imaging. ACR BI-RADS Atlas, breast imaging reporting and data system. Reston, VA: American College of Radiology; 2013.

29. Narayanan D, Madsen KS, Kalinyak JE, et al. Interpretation of positron emission mammography and MRI by experienced breast imaging radiologists: performance and observer reproducibility. AJR Am J Roentgenol 2011;196(4):971–81.

30. Raylman RR, Majewski S, Weisenberger AG, et al. Positron emission mammography-guided breast biopsy. J Nucl Med 2001;42(6):960–6.

31. Kalinyak JE, Schilling K, Berg WA, et al. PET-guided breast biopsy. Breast J 2011;17(2):143–51.

32. Argus A, Mahoney MC. Positron emission mammography: diagnostic imaging and biopsy on the same day. AJR Am J Roentgenol 2014; 202(1):216–22.

33. Choudhery S, Seiler S. Positron emission mammography imaging with low activity fluorodeoxyglucose and novel utilization in core-needle biopsy sampling. World J Nucl Med 2015;14(1):63–5.

34. Park CKS, Bax JS, Gardi L, et al. Development of a mechatronic guidance system for targeted ultrasound-guided biopsy under high-resolution positron emission mammography localization. Med Phys 2021;48(4):1859–73.

35. Hellingman D, Teixeira SC, Donswijk ML, et al. A novel semi-robotized device for high-precision (18)F-FDG-guided breast cancer biopsy. Rev Esp Med Nucl Imagen Mol 2017;36(3):158–65.

36. Caldarella C, Treglia G, Giordano A. Diagnostic performance of dedicated positron emission mammography using fluorine-18-fluorodeoxyglucose in women with suspicious breast lesions: a meta-analysis. Clin Breast Cancer 2014;14(4):241–8.

37. Keshavarz K, Jafari M, Lotfi F, et al. Positron emission mammography (PEM) in the diagnosis of breast cancer: a systematic review and economic evaluation. Med J Islam Repub Iran 2020;34:100.

38. Sueoka S, Sasada S, Masumoto N, et al. Performance of dedicated breast positron emission tomography in the detection of small and low-grade breast cancer. Breast Cancer Res Treat 2021; 187(1):125–33.

39. Sasada S, Kimura Y, Masumoto N, et al. Breast cancer detection by dedicated breast positron emission tomography according to the World Health Organization classification of breast tumors. Eur J Surg Oncol 2021;47(7):1588–92.

40. de Andrés Gómez A, Villalba Ferrer F, Ferrer Rebolleda J, et al. Correlation between MAMMI-PET findings and anatomopathological outcomes in breast cancer patients. Nucl Med Commun 2022;43(10):1058–66.

41. Hashimoto R, Akashi-Tanaka S, Watanabe C, et al. Diagnostic performance of dedicated breast positron emission tomography. Breast Cancer 2022;29(6):1013–21.

42. Nakamoto R, Nakamoto Y, Ishimori T, et al. Diagnostic performance of a novel dedicated breast PET scanner with C-shaped ring detectors. Nucl Med Commun 2017;38(5):388–95.

43. Dai D, Song X, Wang M, et al. Comparison of diagnostic performance of three-dimensional positron emission mammography versus whole body positron emission tomography in breast cancer. Contrast Media Mol Imaging 2017;2017:5438395.

44. Berg WA, Madsen KS, Schilling K, et al. Breast cancer: comparative effectiveness of positron emission mammography and MR imaging in presurgical planning for the ipsilateral breast. Radiology 2011; 258(1):59–72.

45. Nishimatsu K, Nakamoto Y, Miyake KK, et al. Higher breast cancer conspicuity on dbPET compared to WB-PET/CT. Eur J Radiol 2017;90:138–45.

46. Schilling K, Narayanan D, Kalinyak JE, et al. Positron emission mammography in breast cancer presurgical planning: comparisons with magnetic resonance imaging. Eur J Nucl Med Mol Imaging 2011;38(1): 23–36.

47. Sasada S, Masumoto N, Goda N, et al. Which type of breast cancers is undetectable on ring-type dedicated breast PET? Clin Imaging 2018;51:186–91.

48. Berg WA, Weinberg IN, Narayanan D, et al. High-resolution fluorodeoxyglucose positron emission tomography with compression ("positron emission mammography") is highly accurate in depicting primary breast cancer. Breast J 2006;12(4):309–23.

49. Berg WA, Madsen KS, Schilling K, et al. Comparative effectiveness of positron emission mammography and MRI in the contralateral breast of women with newly diagnosed breast cancer. AJR Am J Roentgenol 2012;198(1):219–32.

50. Hunt KN, Swanson T, O'Connor MK, et al. Detection of multicentric breast cancer using dedicated breast PET. Breast J 2019;25(3):512–4.

51. Slanetz PJ, Moy L, Baron P, et al. ACR Appropriateness Criteria((R)) monitoring response to neoadjuvant systemic therapy for breast cancer. J Am Coll Radiol 2017;14(11s):S462–s475.

52. Soldevilla-Gallardo I, Medina-Ornelas SS, Villarreal-Garza C, et al. Usefulness of positron emission mammography in the evaluation of response to neoadjuvant chemotherapy in patients with breast cancer. Am J Nucl Med Mol Imaging 2018;8(5):341–50.

53. Jones EF, Ray KM, Li W, et al. Dedicated breast positron emission tomography for the evaluation of early response to neoadjuvant chemotherapy in breast cancer. Clin Breast Cancer 2017;17(3): e155–9.

54. Noritake M, Narui K, Kaneta T, et al. Evaluation of the response to breast cancer neoadjuvant chemotherapy using 18F-FDG positron emission

mammography compared with whole-body 18F-FDG PET: a prospective observational study. Clin Nucl Med 2017;42(3):169–75.

55. Koyasu H, Goshima S, Noda Y, et al. The feasibility of dedicated breast PET for the assessment of residual tumor after neoadjuvant chemotherapy. Jpn J Radiol 2019;37(1):81–7.

56. Sasada S, Masumoto N, Goda N, et al. Dedicated breast PET for detecting residual disease after neoadjuvant chemotherapy in operable breast cancer: a prospective cohort study. Eur J Surg Oncol 2018; 44(4):444–8.

57. Tokuda Y, Yanagawa M, Fujita Y, et al. Prediction of pathological complete response after neoadjuvant chemotherapy in breast cancer: comparison of diagnostic performances of dedicated breast PET, whole-body PET, and dynamic contrast-enhanced MRI. Breast Cancer Res Treat 2021;188(1):107–15.

58. Masumoto N, Kadoya T, Sasada S, et al. Intratumoral heterogeneity on dedicated breast positron emission tomography predicts malignancy grade of breast cancer. Breast Cancer Res Treat 2018; 171(2):315–23.

59. Sakaguchi R, Kataoka M, Kanao S, et al. Distribution pattern of FDG uptake using ring-type dedicated breast PET in comparison to whole-body PET/CT scanning in invasive breast cancer. Ann Nucl Med 2019;33(8):570–8.

60. Sasada S, Shiroma N, Goda N, et al. The relationship between ring-type dedicated breast PET and immune microenvironment in early breast cancer. Breast Cancer Res Treat 2019;177(3):651–7.

61. Graña-López L, Herranz M, Domínguez-Prado I, et al. Can dedicated breast PET help to reduce overdiagnosis and overtreatment by differentiating between indolent and potentially aggressive ductal carcinoma in situ? Eur Radiol 2020;30(1):514–22.

62. Graña-López L, Herranz M, Domínguez-Prado I, et al. Dedicated breast PET value to evaluate BI-RADS 4 breast lesions. Eur J Radiol 2018;108: 201–7.

63. Bitencourt AG, Lima EN, Macedo BR, et al. Can positron emission mammography help to identify clinically significant breast cancer in women with suspicious calcifications on mammography? Eur Radiol 2017;27(5):1893–900.

64. Malhotra A, Tincey S, Naidu V, et al. Characterisation of MRI indeterminate breast lesions using dedicated breast PET and prone FDG PET-CT in patients with breast cancer-A Proof-of-Concept study. J Pers Med 2020;10(4).

65. Weinstein SP, Slanetz PJ, Lewin AA, et al. ACR Appropriateness Criteria® supplemental breast cancer screening based on breast density. J Am Coll Radiol 2021;18(11s):S456–s473.

66. Yamamoto Y, Tasaki Y, Kuwada Y, et al. A preliminary report of breast cancer screening by positron emission mammography. Ann Nucl Med 2016; 30(2):130–7.

67. Macdonald LR, Wang CL, Eissa M, et al. Positron emission mammography (PEM): effect of activity concentration, object size, and object contrast on phantom lesion detection. Med Phys 2012;39(10): 6499–508.

68. MacDonald LR, Hippe DS, Bender LC, et al. Positron emission mammography image interpretation for reduced image count levels. J Nucl Med 2016; 57(3):348–54.

69. Satoh Y, Sekine T, Omiya Y, et al. Reduction of the fluorine-18-labeled fluorodeoxyglucose dose for clinically dedicated breast positron emission tomography. EJNMMI Phys 2019;6(1):21.

70. Satoh Y, Imai M, Ikegawa C, et al. Image quality evaluation of real low-dose breast PET. Jpn J Radiol 2022;40(11):1186–93.

71. Fujioka T, Satoh Y, Imokawa T, et al. Proposal to improve the image quality of short-acquisition time-dedicated breast positron emission tomography using the pix2pix generative adversarial network. Diagnostics 2022;12(12):3114.

72. Teixeira SC, Rebolleda JF, Koolen BB, et al. Evaluation of a hanging-breast PET system for primary tumor visualization in patients with stage I-III breast cancer: comparison with standard PET/CT. AJR Am J Roentgenol 2016;206(6):1307–14.

73. Iima M, Nakamoto Y, Kanao S, et al. Clinical performance of 2 dedicated PET scanners for breast imaging: initial evaluation. J Nucl Med 2012;53(10): 1534–42.

74. O'Connor MK, Tran TD, Swanson TN, et al. Improved visualization of breast tissue on a dedicated breast PET system through ergonomic redesign of the imaging table. EJNMMI Res 2017;7(1):100.

75. Samanta S, Jiang J, Hamdi M, et al. Performance comparison of a dedicated total breast PET system with a clinical whole-body PET system: a simulation study. Phys Med Biol 2021;66(11). https://doi.org/10.1088/1361-6560/abfb16.

76. Polemi AM, Kogler AK, Rehm PK, et al. Characterization and pilot Human trial of dedicated breast ring positron emission tomography (BRPET) system. Instruments 2021;5(3):30.

77. Kumar R, Loving VA, Chauhan A, et al. Potential of dual-time-point imaging to improve breast cancer diagnosis with (18)F-FDG PET. J Nucl Med 2005; 46(11):1819–24.

78. Mavi A, Urhan M, Yu JQ, et al. Dual time point 18F-FDG PET imaging detects breast cancer with high sensitivity and correlates well with histologic subtypes. J Nucl Med 2006;47(9):1440–6.

79. Satoh Y, Motosugi U, Imai M, et al. Evaluation of image quality at the detector's edge of dedicated breast positron emission tomography. EJNMMI Phys 2021;8(1):5.

80. Satoh Y, Imai M, Ikegawa C, et al. Effect of radioactivity outside the field of view on image quality of dedicated breast positron emission tomography: preliminary phantom and clinical studies. Ann Nucl Med 2022;36(12):1010–8.

81. Yuge S, Miyake KK, Ishimori T, et al. Reproducibility assessment of uptake on dedicated breast PET for noise discrimination. Ann Nucl Med 2023;37(2): 121–30.

82. Moscoso A, Ruibal Á, Domínguez-Prado I, et al. Texture analysis of high-resolution dedicated breast (18) F-FDG PET images correlates with immunohistochemical factors and subtype of breast cancer. Eur J Nucl Med Mol Imaging 2018;45(2):196–206.

83. Hathi DK, Li W, Seo Y, et al. Evaluation of primary breast cancers using dedicated breast PET and whole-body PET. Sci Rep 2020;10(1):21930.

84. Satoh Y, Hirata K, Tamada D, et al. Texture analysis in the diagnosis of primary breast cancer: comparison of high-resolution dedicated breast positron emission tomography (dbPET) and whole-body PET/CT. Front Med 2020;7:603303.

85. Satoh Y, Tamada D, Omiya Y, et al. Diagnostic performance of the support vector machine model for breast cancer on ring-shaped dedicated breast PET images. J Comput Assist Tomogr 2020;44(3): 413–8.

86. Cheng J, Ren C, Liu G, et al. Development of high-resolution dedicated PET-based radiomics machine learning model to Predict axillary lymph node status in early-stage breast cancer. Cancers 2022;14(4).

87. Jones EF, Ray KM, Li W, et al. Initial experience of dedicated breast PET imaging of ER+ breast cancers using [F-18]fluoroestradiol. NPJ Breast Cancer 2019;5:12.

88. Thakur ML, Zhang K, Berger A, et al. VPAC1 receptors for imaging breast cancer: a feasibility study. J Nucl Med 2013;54(7):1019–25.

89. Dehdashti F, Wu N, Ma CX, et al. Association of PET-based estradiol-challenge test for breast cancer progesterone receptors with response to endocrine therapy. Nat Commun 2021;12(1):733.

90. Fowler A, Salem K, Henze Bancroft L, et al. Targeting the progesterone receptor in breast cancer using simultaneous FFNP breast PET/MRI: a pilot study. J Nucl Med 2022;63(Supplement 2):2589.

91. Ulaner GA, Hyman DM, Lyashchenko SK, et al. 89Zr-Trastuzumab PET/CT for detection of Human Epidermal Growth Factor receptor 2-positive metastases in patients with Human Epidermal Growth Factor receptor 2-negative primary breast cancer. Clin Nucl Med 2017;42(12):912–7.

92. Carmona-Bozo JC, Manavaki R, Woitek R, et al. Hypoxia and perfusion in breast cancer: simultaneous assessment using PET/MR imaging. Eur Radiol 2021;31(1):333–44.

93. Kostakoglu L, Duan F, Idowu MO, et al. A phase II study of 3'-deoxy-3'-18F-fluorothymidine PET in the assessment of early response of breast cancer to neoadjuvant chemotherapy: results from ACRIN 6688. J Nucl Med 2015;56(11):1681–9.

94. Backhaus P, Burg MC, Roll W, et al. Simultaneous FAPI PET/MRI targeting the fibroblast-activation protein for breast cancer. Radiology 2022;302(1): 39–47.

Potential Clinical Applications of Dedicated Prostate Positron Emission Tomography

Paolo Castellucci, MD*, Riccardo Mei, MD, Andrea Farolfi, MD, Cristina Nanni, MD, Stefano Fanti, MD

KEYWORDS

- Prostate • PET-CT • PSMA • Tomograph • Staging

KEY POINTS

- PET-computed tomography prostate-specific membrane antigen (PSMA) ligands in the detection of prostate cancer (PCa) foci.
- Clinical applications of dedicated PET prostate scanners.
- Detection of PCa foci to address and guide biopsy.
- PCa T staging.
- PCa N staging.

INTRODUCTION

Prostate cancer (PCa) is the most common type of cancer among men in Europe, causing 375,304 deaths in 2020.[1] In case of prostate specific antigen (PSA) increase, usually the first imaging method performed is transrectal ultrasound (TRUS), which has suboptimal accuracy especially for the detection of small cancer foci.[2]

In the last few years, dedicated MRI sequences have been introduced as the imaging of choice to diagnose PCa. European Association of Urology (EAU) in yearly guidelines published in 2022[6] recommends performing MRI in patients at high risk of PCa, according to PSA levels, even before bioptic procedure in order to guide biopsy sites and potentially reduce the number of samples needed to reach a diagnosis of cancer. EAU based this recommendation on the relatively high accuracy showed by MRI in detecting clinically significant PCa (csPCa) foci.

The introduction of PI-RADSv2 (Prostate Imaging–Reporting And Data System) scoring system,[3] reduced interreader reproducibility, and improved MRI's accuracy, which is around 75% to 85% in any of the published series so far.[4]

In the last few years, new prostate-specific radiopharmaceuticals, prostate-specific membrane antigen (PSMA) inhibitors in particular, are making possible a potential use of PET in this setting. PET could be used to enhance the accuracy of MRI in case of inconclusive findings such as the conditions of PI-RADSv2 scores classified as 2 or 3. An attempt to classify the role of PSMA PET findings in patients with high risk for cancer before biopsy has been proposed by Emmett and coauthors.[5] In this series, a 1 to 5 visual score is proposed (PRIMARY score) with the aim of standardizing PSMA PET reading for the detection of intraprostatic cancer foci.

However, standard whole-body-all-purpose PET-CT instruments have a spatial resolution in

Nuclear Medicine, IRCCS Azienda Ospedaliero-Universitaria di Bologna, Bologna, Italy
* Corresponding author. Nuclear Medicine Unit, IRCCS Azienda Ospedaliero-Universitaria di Bologna, Policlinico S.Orsola, Via Massarenti 9, Bologna 40138, Italy.
E-mail address: paolo.castellucci@aosp.bo.it

PET Clin 19 (2024) 119–124
https://doi.org/10.1016/j.cpet.2023.09.003

the range of 4 to 6 mm, making difficult the detection and precise localization of small cancer lesions. Therefore, to increase the sensitivity of standard PET tomographs in the detection of intraprostatic foci, adoption of dedicated acquisition protocols including full-dose CT and longer acquisition time or delayed or dynamic images acquisition may enhance the role of this modality in this setting.[6]

Theoretically, a dedicated prostate PET/CT tomograph could improve the sensitivity of PET as well as the spatial resolution, which may allow fusion images with MRI and TRUS and reduce the number of inconclusive biopsies performed. The reduction of the number of biopsies needed to reach a final diagnosis of PCa might also have a significant influence on reducing well-known adverse events that could occur after saturation biopsies.[7]

A dedicated PET instrument could reduce the number of random biopsies performed, the time spent, patient discomfort, and the incidence of complications.[8]

The other potential domain of application will include an accurate T staging of PCa.

In this research, MRI plays a role in the detection of extracapsular invasion and seminal vesicle invasion (SVI) with limited role in the detection of lymph node metastatic spread. The addiction of high-resolution PET images to MRI could increase the diagnostic accuracy of both methods leading to a better T stage classification and consequently to an optimized patient management.[9]

Finally, a better definition of N status (N0-N1 vs N2) could help surgeons and/or radiation oncologist in the decision-making process for an optimal approach to the primary treatment of these patients.[2]

The aim of this scientific communication is to present the potential value of a dedicated PET tomograph in the management of patients with PCa and to review the literature and report the attempts that have been made in such initiatives.

STATE OF THE ART OF THE DETECTION OF PROSTATE CANCER FOCI

PSA testing and transrectal random biopsies have been, for decades, the standard approach for the diagnosis of PCa. Ultrasound-guided biopsies can be performed via transrectal (TR-US) or via transperineal procedures.[10] This approach however results in overdiagnosis of insignificant cancers, missing clinically significant malignancies, and biopsy-related morbidity.[11,12]

Nowadays, MRI is the imaging modality of choice to localize suspicious areas that could be targeted by guided biopsies.[2,13] However, the accuracy of MRI imaging in the detection and characterization

of clinically significant cancer foci (csPCa) is suboptimal, leading to certain morbidities and delay in the diagnosis.[14–16] A meta-analysis of this approach revealed a pooled sensitivity of 0.91 (95% CI 0.83–0.95) and a pooled specificity of 0.37 (95% CI 0.29–0.46) in patients presenting International Society of Urological Pathology (ISUP) grade greater than 2.[17] Interestingly, in the same study, the accuracy of MRI did not increase significantly when only cancers with ISUP grade greater than 3, were selected for the analysis.

Therefore, MRI should be performed in patients with high suspicious of PCa based on PSA values, TRUS, digital rectal exploration, and other clinical features[2] as the first imaging modality before biopsy. However, this method is not very accurate so the clinicians will welcome any other imaging that could provide complementary information.

POSITRON EMISSION TOMOGRAPHY IN THE DETECTION OF PROSTATE CANCER

The first attempts to determine the accuracy of PET in the detection of intraprostatic cancer foci was made by ^{11}C-Choline PET/CT[18] with promising results. Farsad and colleagues showed a sensitivity, specificity, accuracy, positive predictive value (PPV), and negative predictive value (NPV) were 66%, 81%, 71%, 87%, and 55%, respectively.

In recent years, with the wide spread availability of ^{68}Ga-labeled or ^{18}F-labeled PSMA radiopharmaceuticals for assessing PCa has enhanced the role of PET for detecting the presence of intraprostatic cancer because PSMA is overexpressed in the majority of prostatic cancer histotypes.[19] Moreover, PSMA expression is mostly related to the Gleason score.[20]

We should emphasize that in addition to PSMA-based PET radiopharmaceuticals, promising results have been also achieved using ^{68}Ga-RM2 for the detection of cancer foci suitable for focal treatment by high-intensity focused ultrasound (HIFU).[21]

An attempt to standardize PSMA PET reading for patients at presentation before biopsy has been proposed by experienced Australian team.[5] This prospective multicenter phase II imaging trial enrolled men with suspected PCa with no earlier biopsy, and a recent mpMRI examination. The study enrolled 291 men who underwent MRI, ^{68}Ga-PSMA PET/CT, and systematic biopsy with or without targeted biopsy. MRI was read using PI-RADSv2 and PSMA PET separately using PRIMARY score 1 to 5. Of the 291 men enrolled, 162 (56%) showed csPCa according to histopathological analysis. Summarizing, sensitivity, specificity, PPV, and NPV for low-risk features at ^{68}Ga-PSMA PET/CT (PRIMARY score = 1–3) versus high-risk features at ^{68}Ga-PSMA PET/CT (PRIMARY score = 4–5) were 88%, 64%, 76%, and 81% respectively. For MRI these values were 83%, 53%, 69%, and 72%, respectively (PI-RADSv2 score = 2 vs 3–5).

Authors correctly conclude that the use of PRIMARY score incorporating intraprostatic pattern and intensity on ^{68}Ga-PSMA PET/CT shows high diagnostic accuracy for csPCa and could be used in addiction to MRI as a complementary imaging method. Recently, the same group published data about synchronous or independent reading of MRI/PSMA-PET. They concluded that the synchronous reading of MRI and PET/CT slightly improves reader certainty. However, independent reading of PSMA-PET and MRI provided similar diagnostic performance to synchronous PSMA-PET/MRI reads.[22,23]

POSITRON EMISSION TOMOGRAPHY IN THE T STAGING OF PROSTATE CANCER

The role of PSMA PET for determining tumor T stage in PCa is not well established at this institution.

In a meta-analysis[9] that included 27 studies (4 studies with PET/MRI and 23 studies with PSMA PET/CT, for a total of 1901 patients enrolled), the authors demonstrated that the diagnostic accuracy of 68Ga-PSMA PET in association with MRI, measured as the pooled natural logarithm of diagnostic odds ratio, for the detection of extracapsular extension (ECE) was 2.27 (95% CI 1.21–3.32). Although for SVI, it was 3.50 (95% CI 2.14–4.86). For PET/CT, only these values were 2.45 (95% CI 0.75–4.14) and 2.94 (95% CI 2.26–3.63), respectively. However, for ^{68}Ga-PSMA PET/CT only, the diagnostic accuracy for ECE was 2.45 (95% CI 0.75–4.14). These results suggest comparable diagnostic accuracy between PET/CT and PET/MRI with wide and overlapping ranges.

In conclusion, the potential added value of PET for T staging (detection of extracapsular or SVI) is still unclear because results are largely influenced by patient population selected for these early trials. As such, the role of a dedicated PET tomograph is unclear and would require further investigation.

POSITRON EMISSION TOMOGRAPHY IN THE N STAGING OF PROSTATE CANCER

An accurate nodal staging before primary treatment is essential for managing patients with PCa at presentation.

At this juncture, many articles have been published in the last few years describing a suboptimal sensitivity but high specificity in the detection of nodal metastasis for PET PSMA, when performed in high-risk or unfavorable intermediate-risk patients.[24,25] The first randomized trial published in 2021 by Hoffmann and colleagues showed high accuracy of PSMA PET in the detection of N metastatic spread when compared with standard CT staging.[26] The limitation of PSMA PET is related to the size of the metastatic lesions in the lymph nodes because of suboptimal spatial resolution of standard PET instruments. In a large series of patients treated with salvage Lymph Node dissection (2292 removed), Abufaraj and colleagues[27] found that the median diameter of detectable lesions in the positive lymph nodes on PSMA PET was 7.2 mm, whereas that of negative scans was 3.4 mm. These data have been confirmed in many other series[24,25] and indicate that the size of metastatic spread in the lymph node is the main factor influencing the sensitivity of PET imaging in this setting. A dedicated tomograph with higher spatial resolution could enhance the role of PET in staging patients with PCa.

CURRENT COMMERCIALLY AVAILABLE PET/CT TOMOGRAPHS

Currently, the spatial resolution of the majority of PET scanners in the market is in the range of 3 to 5 mm. However, it is known that most metastatic lesions are much smaller in size. Therefore, a dedicated PET scanner with a high spatial resolution will be ideal for such settings. Despite many technical difficulties in designing and building a dedicated PET tomograph for this purpose, a team of Physicists from University of Valencia in Spain lead by prof A.J. Gonzales has successfully built an in-house prototype and described its performance in the literature.[28] In this review, we describe the characteristics of the ProsPET Scanner.

THE DEDICATED POSITRON EMISSION TOMOGRAPHY (ProsPET) TOMOGRAPH

Cañizares and colleagues[28] have designed and assembled a novel dedicated PET scanner, named Pros PET, for assessing patients with suspected PCa. ProsPET has an aperture of about 410 mm in diameter, and its ring includes 24 detector blocks separated by a thin gap of 4 mm. Each one of the 24 detector modules of the ProsPET is based on a single monolithic LYSO scintillation crystal of $50 \times 50 \times 15$ mm^3. The transaxial field of view (FOV) is about 300 mm while axial FOV is about 46 mm. However, the axial FOV can be increased to about 80 mm by displacing the ring and allowing image overlapping. The system has 2 movable parts that open and close with an accuracy of about 0.5 mm to ease patient positioning. The system's full width at half maximum is less than 2 mm for all positions, except the radial component that increases to about 2.5 mm at the very edge of the FOV.

The construction and commercialization of a PET instrument dedicated to imaging the prostate gland potentially may have a significant influence in selected patient settings as follows:

1. The most clinically relevant application for a PET tomograph dedicated to the prostate in combination with MRI is the detection of clinically significant intraprostatic disease in patients at high risk of disease who have not undergone biopsy. In this setting, the high accuracy of the PSMA PET/CT (along with findings on MRI) could lead to image-guided biopsies of suspected lesions. There are several image-merging software available capable of fusing MRI and PET images on TRUS images.[29,30] This could lead to significant saving of time and morbidity (reduced number of biopsies performed). This approach will enhance the diagnostic accuracy by making diagnosis possible only by performing a few targeted biopsies on the suspected lesions on images generated by this instrument.[12]

2. A better definition of the presence, the location and the size of intraprostatic cancer site could have beneficial outcomes not only for successful biopsy but also in the treatment of cancer in patients with low-to-intermediate risk eligible for focal therapies such as HIFU (21) brachytherapy or other focal therapies such as cryo-ablation, photodynamic therapy, microwave-coagulation, electroporation, and laser ablation.[31]

3. This instrument could increase the T staging accuracy in patients with high-risk disease without evidence of distant metastatic lesions by the existing modalities. In particular, it could provide useful information on the invasion of the capsule (ie, the detection of the extraprostatic spread of the disease) and seminal vesicles invasion. It could also assess the invasion of the nearby structures such as bladder-rectum. Future research should focus on head-to-head comparison of PSMA and MRI to investigate if either one has additional value in T staging.

SUMMARY

The clinical utility of a dedicated PET tomograph to examine the prostate gland could be of great value to assess high-risk patients in the prebiopsy setting in association with the information provided by MRI in order to reduce the number of bioptic samples needed to reach a final diagnosis. It could better define the location, number, and size of neoplastic sites in intermediate-risk patients eligible for focal therapies. Furthermore, in association with the information provided by the MRI, it could better define the state of the primary disease and presence of extracapsular localizations. Finally, this imaging modality could increase the accuracy of N staging in this common and potentially fatal malignancy.

FUNDING

This research received no external funding.

ACKNOWLEDGMENTS

Substantial contributions to the conception or design of the work by P. Castellucci, R. Mei, A. Farolfi, C. Nanni; Drafting the work or revising it critically for important intellectual content by P. Castellucci, R. Mei, A. Farolfi, and C. Nanni. Final approval of the version to be published P. Castellucci, R. Mei, A. Farolfi, C. Nanni, and S. Fanti. Agreement to be accountable for all aspects of the study in ensuring that questions related to the accuracy or integrity of any part of the study are appropriately investigated and resolved.

DISCLOSURE

The authors: P. Castellucci, R. Mei, A. Farolfi, C. Nanni have nothing to disclose. S. Fanti is Honorarium/Speakers Bureau/Consultancy for AAA, Astellas, Amgen, Bayer, Debio, GE, Janssen, Novartis, Telix.

REFERENCES

1. GLOBOCAN 2020. Available at: https://gco.iarc.fr/today/data/factsheets/cancers/27-Prostate-fact-sheet.pdf/datasources-methods. Accessed 30 January 2023.

2. EAU Pocket Guidelines. edn presented at the EAU Annual Congress Amsterdam 2022. ISBN 978-94-92671-16-5.

3. Turkbey B, Rosenkrantz AB, Haider MA, et al. Prostate imaging reporting and data system version 2.1: 2019 Update of prostate imaging reporting and data system version 2. Eur Urol 2019;76(3):340–51. https://doi.org/10.1016/j.eururo.2019.02.033.

4. Westphalen AC, McCulloch CE, Anaokar JM, et al. Variability of the positive predictive value of PI-RADS for prostate MRI across 26 centers: experience of the society of abdominal radiology prostate cancer disease focused panel. Radiology 2020;296:76–84.

5. Emmett L, Papa N, Buteau J. The PRIMARY score: using intraprostatic ^{68}Ga-PSMA PET/CT patterns to

optimize prostate cancer diagnosis. J Nucl Med 2022;63(11):1644–50.

6. Yang DM, Li F, Bauman G, et al. Kinetic analysis of dominant intraprostatic lesion of prostate cancer using quantitative dynamic [^{18}F]DCFPyL-PET: comparison to [^{18}F]fluorocholine-PET. EJNMMI Res 2021;11(1):2.

7. Ferraro DA, Becker AS, Kranzbühler B. Diagnostic performance of ^{68}Ga-PSMA-11 PET/MRI-guided biopsy in patients with suspected prostate cancer: a prospective single-center study. Eur J Nucl Med Mol Imaging 2021;48(10):3315–24.

8. Papagiannopoulos D, Abern M, Wilson N, et al. Predictors of infectious complications after targeted prophylaxis for prostate needle biopsy. J Urol 2018;199:155–60.

9. Ling SW, de Jong AC, Schoots IG, et al. Comparison of ^{68}Ga-labeled prostate-specific membrane antigen ligand positron emission tomography/magnetic resonance imaging and positron emission tomography/Computed tomography for primary staging of prostate cancer: a systematic review and meta-analysis. Eur Urol Open Sci 2021;33:61–71.

10. Power J, Murphy M, Hutchinson B, et al. Transperineal ultrasound-guided prostate biopsy: what the radiologist needs to know Insights Imaging 2022; 13(1):77.

11. Sosenko A, Owens RG, Yang AL, et al. Non-infectious complications following transrectal prostate needle biopsy - outcomes from over 8000 procedures. Prostate Int 2022;10(3):158–61.

12. Brassil M, Li Y, Ordon M, et al. Infection complications after transrectal ultrasound-guided prostate biopsy: a radiology department's experience and strategy for improvement. Can Urol Assoc J 2022; 16(11):E523–7.

13. Rouviere O, Puech P, Renard-Penna R, et al. Use of prostate systematic and targeted biopsy on the basis of multiparametric MRI in biopsy-naïve patients (MRI-FIRST): a prospective, multicentre, paired diagnostic study. Lancet Oncol 2019;20:100–9.

14. Dell'Oglio P, Stabile A, Soligo M, et al. There is no way to avoid systematic prostate biopsies in addition to multiparametric magnetic resonance imaging targeted biopsies. Eur Urol Oncol 2020;3: 112–8.

15. Elkhoury FF, Felker ER, Kwan L, et al. Comparison of targeted vs systematic prostate biopsy in men who are biopsy naive: the prospective assessment of image registration in the diagnosis of prostate cancer (PAIREDCAP) study. JAMA Surg 2019; 154:811–8.

16. Lahoud J, Doan P, Kim LH, et al. Transperineal systematic biopsies in addition to targeted biopsies are important in the detection of clinically significant prostate cancer. ANZ J Surg 2021;91:584–9.

17. Drost FJH, Osses DF, Nieboer D, et al. Prostate MRI, with or without MRI-targeted biopsy, and systematic biopsy for detecting prostate cancer. Cochrane Database Syst Rev 2019;4:CD012663.

18. Farsad M, Schiavina R, Castellucci P, et al. Detection and localization of prostate cancer: correlation of (11)C-choline PET/CT with histopathologic step-section analysis. J Nucl Med 2005 Oct;46(10):1642.

19. Paschalis A, Sheehan B, Riisnaes R, et al. Prostate-specific membrane antigen heterogeneity and DNA repair defects in prostate cancer. Eur Urol 2019;76: 469–78.

20. Ferda J, Hes O, Hora M, et al. Assessment of prostate carcinoma aggressiveness: relation to ^{68}Ga-PSMA-11-PET/MRI and Gleason score. Anticancer Res 2023 Jan;43(1):449–53.

21. Duan H, Ghanouni P, Daniel B, et al. A Pilot study of ^{68}Ga-PSMA11 and ^{68}Ga-RM2 PET/MRI for evaluation of prostate cancer Response to high intensity focused ultrasound (HIFU) therapy. J Nucl Med 2022;264783. jnumed.122.

22. Doan P, Counter W, Papa N. Synchronous vs independent reading of prostate-specific membrane antigen positron emission tomography (PSMA-PET) and magnetic resonance imaging (MRI) to improve diagnosis of prostate cancer. BJU Int 2022. https://doi.org/10.1111/bju.15929.

23. Ferraro DA, Hötker AM, Becker, et al. ^{68}Ga-PSMA-11 PET/MRI versus multiparametric MRI in men referred for prostate biopsy: primary tumour localization and interreader agreement. Eur J Hybrid Imaging 2022; 6(1):14.

24. Perera M, Papa N, Roberts M, et al. Gallium-68 prostate-specific membrane antigen positron emission tomography in advanced prostate cancer-updated diagnostic utility, sensitivity, specificity, and Distribution of prostate-specific membrane antigen-avid lesions: a systematic review and meta-analysis. Eur Urol 2020;77(4):403–17. Epub 2019 Feb 14. PMID: 30773328.

25. Mattana F, Muraglia L, Raiwa P, et al. Metastatic sites' location and impact on patient management after the introduction of prostate-specific membrane antigen positron emission tomography in newly diagnosed and biochemically recurrent prostate cancer: a critical review. European association of Urology young academic urologists prostate cancer working party. Eur Urol Oncol 2023. https://doi.org/10.1016/j.euo.2023.01.014. S2588-9311(23)00033-0.

26. Hofman MS, Lawrentschuk N. Francis RJ Prostate-specific membrane antigen PET-CT in patients with high-risk prostate cancer before curative-intent surgery or radiotherapy (proPSMA): a prospective, randomised, multicentre study. proPSMA Study Group Collaborators. Lancet 2020;395(10231): 1208–16.

27. Abufaraj M, Grubmüller B, Zeitlinger M, et al. Prospective evaluation of the performance of [^{68}Ga] Ga-PSMA-11 PET/CT(MRI) for lymph node staging

in patients undergoing superextended salvage lymph node dissection after radical prostatectomy. Eur J Nucl Med Mol Imaging 2019;46(10):2169–77. https://doi.org/10.1007/s00259 019 04361.

28. Gabriel Cañizares, Gonzalez-Montoro Andrea. Marta Freire et al Pilot performance of a dedicated prostate PET suitable for diagnosis and biopsy guidance. EJNMMI Phys 2020;7(1):38.

29. Zhao CC, Rossi JK, Wysock JS. Systematic review and meta-analysis of Free-Hand and Fixed-Arm spatial Tracking methodologies in software-guided MRI-TRUS fusion prostate biopsy Platforms. Urology 2023;171:16–22.

30. Xie J, Jin C, Liu M, et al. MRI/Transrectal ultrasound fusion-guided targeted biopsy and transrectal ultrasound-guided systematic biopsy for diagnosis of prostate cancer: a systematic review and meta-analysis. Front Oncol 2022;12:880336.

31. Fujihara A, Ukimura O. Focal therapy of localized prostate cancer. Int J Urol 2022;29(11):1254–63.

Printed and bound by CPI Group (UK) Ltd, Croydon, CR0 4YY

03/10/2024

01040367-0006